OF *IT'S ALL ABOUT LOVE*

This book is a generous literary gift. It's a wisdom book for lovers. Lovers whose own lives are owned by devotion to the daily care of the ones whom they love. This is a book of purest prose, easy to read because of John's winsome writing style and hard to read because care is an indispensable and demanding gift of love. Read it and you will be thankful for John's evident honesty. The book needed to be written.

John Murray has authored an insightful, sympathetic, and motivating guide to navigating a journey no one desires. At this moment John is caring for his wife Rita who has disabling Parkinson's. If you are the child, parent, spouse, or friend of someone whose world has been interrupted by a life-altering condition, you will swiftly recognize that John's personal learnings are germane to your realities. Comfortingly relevant.

Dr. Ron Unruh, Author and Artist. Past President
Evangelical Free Churches of Canada..

It's All About Love is a raw, honest, and breathtaking glimpse into the realities of life as a caregiver. John offers a fresh perspective through the lens of love, practical advice, and a sense that you are seen and not forgotten in your struggles. If you are a caregiver or know someone who is, this book will be a healing balm to those with a hurting heart.

Holly Guy, Coach and Writer at Wholeness Haven, VA, USA..

If you have ever felt alone in your caregiving journey, you won't after reading John Murray's **It's All About Love**. Written from the heart, with honesty and authenticity, John describes the many facets of caring for a loved one with a progressive and debilitating illness. It takes you from the lighter moments of being able to laugh together about the "debacles" that occur, to the sacredness of a "calling" as a Caregiver.

The author aptly conveys the feelings of overwhelm and helplessness in wanting to protect his loved one from the ravages of the disease. As you read, you will find the encouragement you need to "keep on keeping on" and know that there are others who see your heart and understand the complexities that you are dealing with.

Deborah Harrison, MSW (retired), Volunteer Support Group Facilitator for Parkinson's Society of British Columbia, Canada.

In their 60th year of marriage, John Murray finds himself the caregiver to Rita, his Parkinson-stricken wife, and this book is his deeply personal reflection on what this means for them both.

With a sensitive transparency, John Murray explores the progress from diagnosis to acceptance and ongoing struggles as he and his wife cope with an increasing disability. John openly acknowledges his fears, discouragements, and frustrations, but his reflections are always undergirded by a resolute trust in God's loving and providential care. It's All About Love is a beautiful story of marital love and faithfulness expressed in sickness and in health, for better or for worse.

Canada's aging population ensures that the Murray's story will be experienced in many families. John's realistic yet hope-filled study not only helps us understand the unique challenges of caregiving but will encourage those already involved to persevere, as well as help prepare those who will one day find themselves caregivers.

I heartily recommend this timely and loving expression of what true marital love means.

David Daniels, Fellowship Baptist Pastor
& Freelance Writer.

John is a new friend, met on-line in connection with our shared experience of caring for a spouse with Parkinson's. And what a friend, about my age, and like his earlier books so sympathetic and encouraging! With this one he has done it again, another charmer, providing a realistic picture of the caregiving task, including the pain of role-reversal.

His courage and stickability in the face of Rita's extreme
physical disabilities will surely encourage many out
of self-pity, defeat, even despair into true love and
high achievement. May this book be widely used,
for God's glory and the good of many readers..

Priscilla Diana Maryon Turner, BA, MA Cantab., MA, DPhil
Oxon., ODNW, Author of O *LOVE HOW DEEP: A Tale of Three*
Souls* ..

John Murray has done an excellent job of spelling out
the realities of caregiving, the difficulties as well as the
joys. I was moved by the book, so many emotions arose.
As a former 24/7 caregiver to my wife, I can readily
identify with all that is written here. I believe the author's
strong faith has helped sustain him through this part
of their journey together. This book will be a blessing to
many, particularly those who are spousal caregivers.

David North, M.Ed. Retired Principal,
Lions Gate Christian Academy.

John is an inspiration as he faithfully and patiently
cares for his wife Rita. His positive attitude shines
through in everything he writes. It is obvious that
he sees caregiving as a calling from God, not a
burden or a role he fell into by chance. His book will

inspire other caregivers that their service is never
meaningless or in vain, or that they are alone.

Jennifer Friesen, Pastor to Seniors,
White Rock Baptist Church, Surrey, British Columbia.

John Murray, who in his own words is, "just an
ordinary 82-year-old husband taking care of his
78-year-old wife" Rita, who was diagnosed with
Parkinson's in 2008. John shares their challenging
journey in a humble, straightforward way and offers
general advice and encouragement relevant to other
caregivers regardless of the conditions they face.

I appreciate the author's occasional flashes of
humour and his commitment to respecting Rita's
dignity. He encourages her to do what she can for
herself. Every action she undertakes, even putting
on her glasses, takes a long time. But he says, "we
soon learned that time is not of the essence."

I'm inspired and challenged by the author's motivation.
He cares for Rita because he loves her. They both have a
strong faith, and he believes his role is "a call from God."

Elma Schermenauer is an author of many published books.
They include *YesterCanada: Historical Tales of Mystery and Adventure*
and the 1940s-era Mennonite novel *Consider the Sunflowers*.

Other books by John Murray

Miracles: Coincidence or Divine Intervention

Real Faith: What's at the Heart of the Gospel?

Body Parts and the Invisible You.

Discover Your Hidden Self:
Finding Out who you Really Are!

Information on these books is available at
www.jmurray.ca

It's all about
LOVE

Confessions of a Caregiver

JOHN MURRAY

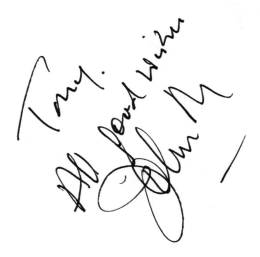

IT'S ALL ABOUT LOVE
Confessions of a Caregiver

Copyright © John Murray, 2021

Published by John Murray, White Rock, Canada

Jacket design: Roger E. Murray
Cover photo: Shutterstock

ISBN 0-978-1-77354-367-3

Publication assistance and digital printing in Canada by

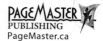
PUBLISHING
PageMaster.ca

To my dear wife Rita, without you there would be no story to tell. By sharing some aspects of your 13-year ordeal with Parkinson's, we hope and pray that many people will be blessed and encouraged

Contents

Introduction...1

Part One - Our Story...5

   Chapter 1 - How Did We Get Here? 7

   Chapter 2 - Everyday Life 21

   Chapter 3 - What is Required of Me? 39

   Chapter 4 - Is There a Limit? 49

   Chapter 5 - When Should I Get Help?.........................59

   Chapter 6 - Is There a Spiritual Side to This? 67

   Chapter 7 - What About Tomorrow? 77

   Chapter 8 - Love Finds a Way!..................................... 85

Part Two - Your Story 93

   My Fellow Caregivers... 95

   About the Author 118

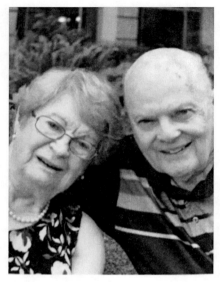

John and Rita Murray on their
59th Wedding Anniversary,
June 30th, 2021

Introduction

I do not reckon myself to be an authority on caregiving. I am just an ordinary 82-year-old husband taking care of his 78-year-old wife. I care for my wife Rita because she is my wife and because I love her. Whether or not I am doing the job right I wouldn't know, but I do know that I am still learning, regardless of the number of years already past.

All I want to do here is to relate how life is and how it has been for us. I plan to share the things that have occurred and affected us on our journey with Parkinson's disease. All illnesses are different, which create different caregiving scenarios. However, certain principles remain the same and interpersonal relationships are similar in these different scenarios. Those who are caregiving will see themselves reflected in our situation and will identify with some of the issues we have faced.

I am fully aware of the many caregivers out there who carry a much heavier load than me, which causes me some reluctance to put pen to paper. However, it has been persuasively suggested by various people that my sharing would be an encouragement to others in a similar situation. Thus, I write in the hope that my experience will be an encouragement to you. A large percentage of caregivers feel alone and discouraged. If you are one of them, I write these words to assure you that you are not alone. If you are struggling, then remember, we are standing with you because many of us are also struggling.

Much has been written on caregiving which is another reason I am reluctant to add anything further, for fear of repetition. However, I simply want to share that which I have discovered along the way in the hope that those who are not caregiving may understand what caring means, so that they might be able to identify with those who are.

Statistics can be cold and meaningless unless you find yourself included in those numbers. The number of people caregiving in North America is staggering – I read it was over 40 million. That seems a huge number, even as an estimate, but I guess with a population of around 400 million in North America, it is quite feasible that 10 percent could be caregiving. There are children looking after aged parents and parents caring for sick children, but I understand that about 60% of all caregiving is spouse caring for spouse.

Although different diseases present different scenarios, caregiving is never easy, regardless of the illness.

I recognize that those people caring for loved ones who are bedridden or have dementia, have a whole different set of procedures from those of us who are dealing with Parkinson's. Although extremely incapacitated the person with Parkinson's normally has some mobility, however small, but does need constant support and care.

Permit me to get something off my chest which I find very disturbing. I am referring to spousal willingness to care. I read that most women "stand by their man" in the event of his illness, whereas a high proportion of men do just the opposite. The ratio is reported to be as high as seven or eight out of ten men abandon their spouses at the onset of a long-term illness. That is extraordinarily high but whatever the ratio, even if it is five out of ten, it makes one almost ashamed of the male sex. It is hard to believe that so many men would ignore their responsibility and bail out from the relationship at such a critical time.

At the very point in life when a wife needs love and support, she is abandoned to take care of herself and often her children as well. Where is the love? How can it suddenly disappear? If there was genuine love before, why would not the illness bring out the love in not wanting to see your loved one suffer? I would have thought every husband would want to do everything he could to alleviate the oncoming suffering as much as possible. It saddens and appalls me to learn this. However, having said this, I am aware that there are millions of men doing an excellent job of caregiving, husbands caring for their spouses and sons caring for parents. So, not all abandon their responsibility. Many have picked up the baton and are running with it.

So, let's think about caregiving. It is not an easy road to travel. In fact, it can be quite difficult at times and often uphill. It is a permanent learning experience. The experience is different for everyone. It's like taking on a job you know nothing about and learn by doing. As you do the same things again and again you quickly pick up the best way, or most efficient way, to do those things.

Dressing and lifting are two daily regular activities, so one learns to be proficient quite quickly. To dress, or even put a coat on someone who cannot bend their arms or assist by cooperating with you, is not without its difficulties and even more so if they are sitting in a wheelchair. One also quickly learns efficient ways to lift. As I lift my wife about twenty-five times a day, bed, chairs, wheelchair, toilet etc., it is necessary to do it the best way possible, without hurting her or me.

But I am getting ahead of myself so let's see how this all started.

Part One

Our Story

CHAPTER 1

How Did We Get Here?

In 1957 I met this kind, considerate, loving, and demure girl. I was soon to discover just how considerate Rita was, being so sensitive to others, putting them first and never wanting to offend. I found out that in her graciousness she usually would give way to the opinions of others before considering her own. But I discovered she was not without opinions and chose to express them when appropriate. For instance, we first met when Rita joined the youth choir of which I was the conductor. She was all of fourteen and I was eighteen. Her first view and opinion of the conductor was that he was "a big-head" and was "too big for his boots!" However, by the time she was fifteen, one year later, she must have changed her mind (maybe she came to her senses!) as we started going out together and four years later, we were married.

Here we are, almost sixty years later with much of the proverbial water having passed under the bridge. As it is for many couples, life has brought its pleasures and its challenges. Over those years Rita has remained the kind, loving and generous person she is. Her generosity, on more than one occasion, would have us giving away more than we could afford, to help others. God blessed us with two children which was one of the pleasures in our marriage. The natural process followed and today we have five grandchildren and two great-grandchildren. We have experienced many happy times, but it has not been without the sad moments as well.

We have both had medical challenges. Our daughter was born with a heart defect and had an operation at 13 weeks old. Rita has experienced several nasty bouts of depression over the years, each lasting about four months. She was also diagnosed with breast cancer in 1986. I had a cancerous tumour removed from the colon in 1984 and then chopped half my thumb off in a lawn-mower accident in 1988. So, we have not been strangers to these and various other medical procedures and adverse medical conditions. However, the on-going situation we face today far outweighs anything we have faced before.

The diagnosis

Rita was diagnosed with Parkinson's Disease in April 2008. When I think back to that time, I cannot remember us being terribly upset or disturbed over what we had just been told. It seems that we simply accepted it for what it was, a doctor's report. Probably it was because the symptoms were seemingly minor and certainly nothing significant to us at that moment. We had no idea of what lay ahead.

This progressive disease of the nervous system initially affected Rita with a small hand tremor, then muscular rigidity and as time has moved on, various other symptoms have occurred, including mobility problems as well as extreme exhaustion. Some years later Rita's diagnosis was changed from pure Parkinson's to Progressive Supra-Nuclear Palsy which, although slightly different, appears to come under the umbrella of Parkinson's as the symptoms are parkinsonian. Unfortunately, we have been informed that there is no specific medicine for PSP, so Rita is treated with the normal Parkinson's medication of Leva-dopa. We, as well as her neurologist, are unsure how effective this is for her condition.

Interestingly two hundred years ago Parkinson's was known as "Palsy."In 1817 Dr James Parkinson wrote an essay on "The Shaking Palsy" and it appears that his name became synonymous with the disease. I read that there are four categories of symptoms with Parkinson's. Regrettably we find that with Rita's tremor, rigidity, freezing, her imbalance and inability to write, she is suffering symptoms from all four categories.

The progression of the disease in Rita has caused a steady decline from walking unaided in 2008, then walking supported by someone else, to the use of a walker and then by 2019 we had to resort to a wheelchair. Today, in 2021, Rita's self-mobility is non-existent, and her balance is virtually zero. She needs constant support from me, from furniture or her walker, although even with the walker she cannot walk unassisted. She can no longer stand on her own.

In her teens Rita was an athlete and enjoyed running. In fact, she still owns medals she won during that time. It is no wonder she has always enjoyed walking. When we had a dog, she was as keen as the dog to get out and walk. Sadly, all that has gone now. There is no more walking except with great difficulty and assistance. However, I am pleased that for the first few years after contracting Parkinson's, Rita showed her determination and kept up her exercise routine to the best of her ability.

She continued with her visits to the women's exercise venue Curves, as in pre-diagnosis days. In fact, Rita completed 800 visits to Curves before finding it too difficult to get in and out of the exercise machines. She then attended a medical exercise clinic where the exercises were customized for Parkinson's patients and people with other incapacitating diseases. After three years, this too had to be abandoned as her balance became too precarious and she was in danger of falling.

So, gradually, over the years since Rita's diagnosis, I have become her full-time caregiver. It was not asked for. It was not sought, but I see it as part of our marriage commitment. She needs assistance in every area of life now and naturally I am the one to give that help. However, I am still her husband first, and caregiver by default.

What is caregiving?

The simplest and most common definition of caregiving is to provide physical and emotional support to those who are unable to care for themselves. But I like to think it is more than that. I believe for me, it is to create the very best environment and the best living conditions so that Rita can fully enjoy life, despite her incapacities. Caregiving is a marathon. It is not a hundred- meter dash. It takes dedication, determination, persistence, and patience. Just like the runner dealing with mental and physical barriers so the caregiver does the same. Hitting the wall of fatigue and exhaustion happens all too frequently but love and concern motivates and drives one on.

The care develops and grows over time, from normal general assistance to ultimately full-time twenty-four-hour attention. For me it all started with small requests of help in areas which had been Rita's domain. For the first several years after the diagnosis, Rita could do the regular chores of housework and meal preparation but gradually that changed. Like other caregivers I started out by doing simple things over the course of a regular day to help and provide support, but then as the disease took hold, Rita's incapacities grew as did the need for help. Slowly it became evident that the daily routine of events was taking its toll and becoming more difficult.

The decline in Rita's abilities and capabilities was hard to accept, for both of us. The helplessness for us to do anything to stop this downward trend was over-whelming and still is today. The physical deterioration in the one you love is heart-wrenching and painful to watch and difficult to handle. I knew Rita always felt bad, if not worse than me, when she was forced to ask for help because of her limitations. Thus, I moved naturally into the full-time caregiver's job.

When you sign up for caregiving you have no idea what it may involve. There are many physical and practi-cal aspects to it as well as the need for regular emotional support. As time passes the same tasks become more regular and often more personal. Nothing is beyond the need for assistance when caring twenty-four-seven for your loved one. Some tasks call for much understanding and patience. What I do for Rita I do because I love her.

To me, Rita's dignity is always critically important. Therefore, as I write I respect Rita's privacy and will always maintain her dignity. She is a very sensitive person, and

I am aware of her thinking and her feelings and respect those too. Hence, I am careful about recounting all the details of our daily activity. So, if I happen to leave a gap or two in my explanations, I hope you will understand. Those of you who are involved in caregiving will readily be able to fill in those gaps. With all illnesses there are situations which are unpleasant to deal with, but such is life as a caregiver. You deal with it and move on. I honestly believe that spouses can do undignified tasks in a dignified way.

Beginning the journey

From the beginning of this Parkinson's journey with Rita, I have tried to get into her shoes, not literally of course, but mentally. I think a lot about the fact that she didn't ask for this situation in which she finds herself. She didn't ask to be where she is. Inwardly she probably dislikes it intensely. Maybe she hates it. She didn't choose it. In fact, she would rather have continued to be independent as she once was, rather than being waited upon. It is certainly not her fault that she needs care. I asked her one day how she felt about being pushed around in a wheelchair. Her reply was "I wish it wasn't so. I wish it didn't have to be!"

How she would love to still be able to dress herself and cook the dinner. How she would prefer to have the ability to do the laundry and iron the clothes, even if there were times earlier in life when those were not her most favourite tasks. Now, in her mind she feels more like a burden, a nuisance, an inconvenience to all around. She is neither a burden nor a nuisance which I try to convey to her. To fully comprehend her situation, I need to theoretically be in her shoes or at least get into her mind. I constantly remind myself of her sense of helplessness and her desire not to be so dependent upon others. At all times, she needs my kindness and understanding. I find that this thinking helps me keep a balanced mental perspective of the overall situation.

It may seem very strange in this modern day for some people to read just how much I had to learn when I started caregiving. Things like cooking, doing the laundry and other household chores. It was simply because we lived in a different age. In that day the role of husband and wife were different from today. I understand that now those responsibilities are shared, and the tasks are not so distinguished by gender. I see this as a good thing because, in the event of a caregiving situation arising in the family like ours, there would be less adjustment to be made by both. Unfortunately for me that was not the case.

I had to become familiar with many things. I quickly learned just how many different aspects of our previous life I had taken for granted. Things which Rita had always handled and undertaken in the house. In all our married life, which to that point had been 50 years, I had never done the laundry. That changed. It grew from just needing my assistance to it being my job. Housework also became too much for Rita so that too dropped into my lap. We did eventually get some help in that area by hiring someone to come in to clean.

Food preparation and cooking was another area of exploration and experimentation for me. I quickly discovered that a boiled egg did not suffice for breakfast, lunch, and dinner. There is something to be said for learning to cook when you are young. Unfortunately, I missed out on that; consequently, I must admit, I came to appreciate ready-made frozen meals. Where was "Skip the Dishes" when I needed it?

Limitations

Accepting of limitations is one of the earliest lessons I learned. It was difficult initially just coming to terms with the fact that your wife has Parkinson's, and that this disease was not going away but in fact will progress and cause her to be more and more incapacitated as time goes by. However, I found the sooner I could accept the situation mentally for what it was, then the sooner I could face it, deal with it, and look for ways to reduce the suffering and concentrate on making life more tolerable for Rita. One could always wish for the things to be different, but it doesn't change the situation. How I have wished that many times.

Recognizing Rita's immobility was one of the first steps in coming to terms with limitations. I could no longer expect her to be able to do the things she previously could, however much she would like to, it was no longer within her capabilities. I discovered how disturbed and frustrated she felt at not being able to help or deal with issues around the home. She hated having to tell me that "such and such needs doing" when normally she would have done it herself. You soon learn that normal everyday activity is no longer normal, and you cannot undertake what used to be a simple everyday activity.

There are other areas of life to which we had to adjust our thinking. No longer could we make a quick trip to the store or go out to our favourite coffee shop. Shopping became a trip out of necessity and not just to browse or window-shop. The time arrives when you realize that going out to church or any other place, has become a major operation. With the indoor preparation of bathroom visits, dressing appropriately, getting into the wheelchair and then the effort of getting into the car, getting out of the car, all presenting different levels of dangers. Such things cause one to think twice about going out once!

The big picture

Gradually you discover that it is more important to take a big picture view of everything. It is so easy to get sidetracked by minimal, inconsequential aspects in the present and allow them to bother you. Looking at the big picture helps you get things in the right and balanced perspective. Little things can get at you if you let them, like if the walker is parked thoughtlessly in the way, or the time taken to throw things away or just putting them down.

With Parkinson's Rita's fingers grip around objects but she cannot freely open them again, so putting a cup down or dropping a tissue into a waste basket takes an inordinate amount of time. The temptation is to jump in, grab the item and deal with it yourself but I try to avoid giving in to that temptation. I find I must let Rita do what she can do for herself. As it is so limited what she can do now, it is wrong to deplete it further just to save a few seconds here or there. In the bigger picture, one asks, what does it matter?

As well as her body not cooperating and increasing immobility, her eyes have also deteriorated. Rita used to be an avid reader. As I write this, I can see four shelves of books which are hers and have brought hours of reading delight to her. Today she cannot get beyond reading a few lines before everything blurs and runs into one.

So, we purchase audible books to which she can listen. Unfortunately, with her constant exhaustion she has the tendency to slip into sleep while the narration continues. I also read to Rita every day. Sometimes in the day or in the evening just before she goes to bed. At this point we have read through nine or ten books.

Another restriction comes in personal care which is particularly hard for a woman. Rita can only wash and do her make-up now. During the pandemic I even became her hairdresser, washing, drying, curling, and combing. Who would have thought, not me! Having hair which looks nice is important to any woman, but I think even more so to Rita, especially when confined to a wheelchair. Looking her best at all times is crucial to me in caring for her. A little combing of the hair and a little make-up goes a long way in making Rita feel more comfortable and acceptable in the company of others. Now I ensure that she is at the hairdressers every week.

I find the progression of the disease in Rita hard to take. Regrettably we know that this is how Parkinson's goes but it makes it no easier for us to accept. The disease has a mind of its own and we can do nothing else but become accustomed to the limitations which have crept up on us over the years. Today Rita needs assistance to make any move. Gratefully it was not always like that. It has been a gradual process, almost imperceptible, except when you compare the situation from year over year, then the comparison is real and concerning.

As caregivers I guess our caring is based either upon duty or love or maybe a little of both. For me I like to think it is love. Naturally there is a responsibility which comes from being married to Rita, but I believe the caring should come from my love and commitment to her. Some might feel they have been landed with the job because there was no one else to step in and I understand that. My experience of caring for my wife comes out of our marriage vows—to me it is all part of the commitment when we uttered the words, "in sickness and in health." Never did we dream how those words might apply down the years. This is the reality of life.

It may be difficult to imagine but caregiving is not all negative. It brings its own rewards. For the most part those cared for appreciate the assistance they receive and recognize the effort expended on their behalf. Gratitude is never far below the surface even if it is not always verbalized. I must admit it is delightful when you hear the words, "Thank you for caring for me!" or "You are the best husband I could have wished for!"

Is caregiving a chore, a challenge, or a privilege? If we are honest, it can be a chore. In fact, it is often hard work. It certainly is a challenge at times, but if we really love the person then it is a privilege. God knew that down the road Rita would need someone to care for her and he has allowed me that privilege and therefore, it has become an honour to care for her and I do it to the best of my ability.

CHAPTER 2

Everyday Life

Although many days look the same and are the same because you have a routine to which you adhere. In fact, often one forgets what day it is because of that continued similarity. However, you can never tell what the day may hold. Two of the needed attitudes to face each day is flexibility and adaptability. Things can change in a moment – and they do. The probability of something going wrong is very high, so if you are too rigid in your thinking, then changes can turn into a major crisis.

Something unexpected happens and your day looks different. Maybe a planned trip to the mall must be abandoned for various reasons. It might be pure exhaustion on Rita's part, and she just doesn't have the energy. Thus, we always remain flexible with plans. This eliminates the element of surprise or concern if we need to make changes. Disappointments come and go. You face them and rise above them. You quickly learn that life is more important than the things that go wrong and the changes which may have to be made.

For us old-timers – I think being in my eighties I qualify for that title – we are familiar with the phrase, "A woman's work is never done!" I can now readily identify with that sentiment and the truth of it. Has it really taken me 59 years of married life to realize that? Probably not, but the present situation has certainly brought it to the foreground.

Rita's principle in housekeeping has always been "Cleanliness is next to Godliness." In other words, she is a "clean freak" which is not said negatively. She just loves to have the place clean and tidy and everything in its place. Even when I tell her that nobody is coming, that makes no difference. Rita hates the place to show any dust but unfortunately, she cannot get up and do the dusting. It seems that I do not have the same observation powers in this regard, so she reminds me of items and places which are not so obvious which need to be dusted, like plants and more obscure walls and baseboards. So, I dust the plants and baseboard because it is important to Rita. However, I don't want to live in a slum either but to me these things are less important compared to Rita's comfort.

What is important?

As I go about the daily tasks of caregiving there is one question which keeps coming to mind "What really is important?" by which I really mean, what should take precedence. Not that anything is unimportant when you are caring for someone but sometimes, I have found it a good thing to prioritize the to-do list.

I admit to occasionally thinking, "Does it have to be done now or can it be done later or even tomorrow?" I know that is procrastination but there are things which under normal circumstances we would have considered important but now they become less so when pressured by time and other things. Issues in the present are usually more significant and important so when time is of the essence, one does think about what can be put off – even knowing Rita would disagree. She tends not to be a pro-crastinator.

There was a time when it bothered me to see food dropped which happens as Rita has difficulty holding her eating utensils, but no longer does it concern me. But again, looking at the big picture I concluded it was a small thing. Things dropped and spilled is no big deal anymore. Messes can be cleaned up. Food can be picked up and clothes can be washed. It is more important that Rita knows that my helping her eat is just another act of love.

In all aspects of my caregiving, I try to bring assistance and support which, in turn, brings her comfort and peace of mind. I place more importance on having Rita know that I am always there for her, whatever the circumstances and whatever time of day or night. This provides Rita with confidence and assurance of my availability for her. I purposely keep this in mind as I have read where those cared for are prone to feel a sense of abandonment and insecurity.

If you are not personally involved in caregiving, some sentences will not adequately convey the real meaning of the activity. For instance, when you read the words, "take someone to the bathroom" it means different things to different people. It would also differ according to the incapacity of the person involved. For us, a short bathroom visit is normally ten to fifteen minutes because it is not just a question of just getting to the bathroom door. It means helping Rita in the bathroom.

Rita's legs freeze up and refuse to move. This is common with Parkinson's patients. This is why it takes so long. The legs stop moving forward and the feet become glued to the floor. It is just as if they have been nailed to the floor. We try going sideways, backwards, or forward – anything to tell the brain we want the feet to move. In their attempt to move forward often the feet will go right up on the toes like a ballerina but still stuck like concrete to the floor. So, once we have moved across the bathroom, we need to change direction to use the facility, which is extremely difficult. Turning is natural for most of us but it is one of the most difficult maneuvers for Parkinson's sufferers. We try different ways to move the legs but for the most part we just must exercise patience and wait for the feet to turn - at the same time trusting there is no urgency in our reason for being there!

Rita's zero balance is not a helpful condition in the bathroom. Holding someone up and attempting to adjust clothing is like being a one-armed paper hanger! When we leave the bathroom, we do everything as before but in reverse. The feet will not turn the way Rita wants them to but with her lack of balance the body tries to go in the desired direction without the legs being ready to move. Hence, all her weight comes my way as I attempt to hold her up by her arms. Getting someone to walk who has virtually zero balance and uncooperating feet is a formidable task. One is constantly aware of the potentiality of falling, which has occurred all too often. A trip to the bathroom seven or eight times a day makes one becomes ultra-sensitive to the potential danger.

It is not dissimilar with showering. The actual showering is fine as we use a stool or shower chair but getting Rita in and out of a one-person shower takes an inordinate amount of time and precision. With the freezing of the feet and legs it takes lots of patience. Occasionally we are forced to abandon the idea for that day. In fact, I have had to reduce the showers from every other day to twice a week because the danger of falling is ever present. If we both fell that could be even more disastrous.

Falls happen

Obviously when Rita has a fall, I am the one to pick her up. For the first few times in the early years of the disease, I put my back out picking her up as she cannot help to get up. It is like lifting dead weight from the floor, and that is never easy. However, I learned by trial and error how to pick her up with less strain on my back and easier for her.

The number of falls which Rita has experienced has always been a concern to me. In fact, at one point I was that concerned at the number of times she had fallen and hit her head, I requested an MRI for Rita from the neurologist. The results came back normal for which we were grateful. We concluded she had a hard head. The rest of her body has also suffered much bruising, particularly her back. I have lived for a while with the expectation of hearing an ominous crash. However, I rarely leave Rita on her own now which helps to eliminate that potentiality.

I remember one particularly bad fall one night. It was 10.50 p.m. Most falls occur in the bathroom, and this was no different. This was in the early days of her disease, so Rita's balance was far better than it is today. She was

standing at the washbasin, lost her balance and fell backwards, crashed through the glass door of the shower, the
shower step and threshold cutting across her back, and
ultimately finished up banging her head on the tiles at
the back of the shower. She came to rest across the floor,
half in and half out of the shower. I lifted her out of the
shower – not an easy task – sat her down, put ice on her
back and head, checked for concussion – no nausea, no
dizziness, she could focus well – decided not to take her
to hospital but kept her awake for another hour before
putting her in bed. Thinking back to it days later, I won-
dered if I should have taken her to the emergency. The
lower portion of her back changed many colours over the
next couple of weeks. That was about 8 years ago.

The one fall which did put her in hospital was at
Thanksgiving 2019. It occurred because Rita was reaching for the light switch, something she was not supposed
to do. She reached out and although she was holding her
walker, she toppled, the walker could not hold her, it
tipped over and she fell out of the bathroom door, hit her
head on the wood floor and immediately her head began
bleeding. The blood was coming out so profusely, like a
tap, I grabbed a towel in an attempt to stop the flow.
While holding the towel in place, I pressed the emergency
button for help and then dialed for the paramedics. Help
came within a short time and Rita was taken by ambu-

lance to the hospital. There she had stiches in her head over her left eye and was kept in overnight.

It was the next morning we ran into a problem. The hospital authorities questioned whether I was competent to care for Rita. After some long discussion they politely said, "You seem to know what you are talking about" which was very kind of them and with that, they allowed me to take Rita home. That is the danger in going to hospital. When it comes time for being released the staff in charge need to know that the patient is going home to adequate care.

We live in a Retirement Community, and it is not uncommon for people to have a fall, maybe break a hip or shoulder, be taken to hospital and not return. Apart from the fact that the injury seems to make them susceptible to pneumonia or some other medical problem, they are often dispatched to some other long term care facility. We want to avoid that at all costs. However, I would never hesitate to call for help or get Rita medical treatment if she needs it. Overall, the hospital situation has caused us to become extremely conscious of potential falls and take appropriate steps to avoid them.

There was one occasion when we both went down together. We were crossing a road, fortunately a side road. This was before Rita used a walker. I was holding her, and she was holding on to me. She stepped off the curb, lost her balance and went down and because she gripped harder as she fell, I went down also. We finished as a heap in the middle of the road. A gentleman rushed out to help us. I got up and we both helped Rita to her feet. We only suffered scrapes and bruises, nothing broken, except our pride took a hit. It could have been worse.

Like many other people with Parkinson's, Rita has sleep issues but not the normal non-sleeping problem. Her difficulty is an inability to move once she lays down. Because of this we ensure Rita is in a comfortable position for the night. As her immobility does not allow her to turn over, she is liable to get bed sores, so I try to create a sleeping environment bearing all this in mind. Also, the Parkinson's causes her head to fall to the left, leaving her with pain in the neck and the back. After many different trials we now have a satisfactory system using six cushions, one pillow, one travelling neck collar and a blanket. This I put together each night and then dismantle again in the morning when I get her up. It seems to work well. She has had no bed sores and the pain in her neck and back have virtually disappeared.

One may put out the light at 11 pm and then hopefully disappear into dreamland until the music wakes you up at 6am. But those hours are by no means sacred. It is not guaranteed that one will remain undisturbed. I sleep with the antennae up just listening for coughing or worse, a choking sound or perhaps just a bathroom call. It is like a mother with her child. A mother can sleep through traffic noise but once her baby utters a sound, she is awake and ready to go. That is the same with caregiving. Night-time visits to the bathroom are the most difficult as one is only half-awake – initially anyway, but once it is all over, one is wide awake and often sleep will become quite elusive.

Enjoying life together

Making memories throughout life is essential and continues to be important during the days of caregiving. Sharing memories is even more important. As we remember days long past and the stories associated with our past life together, it adds meaning and enjoyment to the present. It matters not if the facts are a little hazy. The important thing I find is to share because the stories add flavor to the day. We dig around in the memory box together and discover some happy memories. It is a reminder of places we have been together, of people we have met, and things accomplished. When you have been together for almost sixty years as a married couple there is plenty of material from which to bring up memories of earlier years, of courting days or early marriage days, of our children growing up and their children. Remembering and sharing these stories is good for our mental health. It also adds substance to our discussions and often brings laughter into the arena, which is always a plus.

We enjoy good communication together. Spending time just chatting or discussing some topic of interest or even reading together, brings a semblance of normality into our situation. I am extremely grateful that we do not have to deal with cognitive issues. Rita is mentally competent. She still has her sense of wit and humour but now finds some difficulty in expressing that wit and humour quickly. That aside, we enjoy just spending time together reminiscing.

With Parkinson's the brain is slower in computing questions asked and therefore the reply takes a little longer in coming and sometimes not at all. Rita says that sometimes her exhaustion is so overwhelming that is an effort to talk. I understand that and allow for it in our conversations. However, it does have its downside. When I am in the process of doing something and need Rita's help, like putting clothes on, it is difficult to know what is going on in the mind if there is nothing but silence. I have come to accept that mostly the silence is due to the Parkinson's effect of slowing down the ability to make quick decisions. The brain needs extra time to decide or determine what is the right thing to say, or do, at that moment.

It is difficult to leave Rita now for any length of time, maybe only ten or fifteen minutes at a time. I always make sure she has her emergency call button and knows where I will be and how long I might be out – even if just going to another part of the building. Rita has become my absolute priority – she takes the first place when considering any arrangement.

Being able to get Rita time with other people has been a non-starter during the year and a half of the pandemic. This has been a critical aspect missing from Rita's life. It is crucial and important mentally for Rita to be able to interact with others and not me alone. She needs the stimulation of conversation with other people who think differently to me. She also needs to understand the care and concern that others have for her. She needs to hear what is happening in other people's lives which helps to expand her thinking and helps eliminate her feeling of being boxed in with me. As I write this, it seems that an easing of the pandemic and various protocols that have accompanied it, is in the works. I look forward for Rita's sake to get outside friends in to visit again. Hopefully, that is in place before you read this.

Kindness never goes unnoticed

Kindness on the part of others does not go amiss and unnoticed. Before the pandemic of 2020 came upon us, we attended church every Sunday morning. One of the joys of some Sunday mornings was arriving at the door of the church to find an usher willing and requesting to help with getting Rita into the wheelchair and then taking her inside while I parked the car. It may seem a small insignificant act but to me it was someone reaching out to help. It was most appreciated and expressed to me that others cared and were willing to help.

I find that people watch and take notice of how I care for Rita when in public. On one occasion when we were in another town visiting Rita's brother, who also had Parkinson's, we stopped in a coffee shop for a quick lunch. I got Rita seated at a table and then joined the line to place the order. The lady ahead of me immediately began asking questions about Rita's condition. She informed me that she was a live-in caregiver for a lady in the town there, so she knew something about caring. She indicated how she had watched while I got Rita settled in her chair at the table. Then she promptly said, "I would like to buy lunch for you and your wife." How lovely that was, and I am delighted to say that it has happened more than once. We have been touched and blessed by other people's kindness.

It is amazing the support one feels from such acts of generosity. However, not all people are of similar character. I think of the disapproving looks we have received from other drivers as they have had to drive around my car while I unloaded Rita at a restaurant or hairdressers. They indicate by their looks that an extra thirty seconds involved in that small maneuver is such an encroachment upon their day. They obviously give little thought to the incapacity of the person trying to get in or out of the car. It's unfortunate and sad because one day, they may be in the same position.

I am sure you have heard the phrase, "the new normal." I wonder if there is such a thing for us. I think our new normal is a moving target. New aspects come into play every so often such as more medication or a greater physical difficulty for Rita seems to arise. We accept the changes because we have no other option and move on with our everyday activity. With Rita gradually being able to do less and less, the task grows as time moves on.

In caring and keeping the daily program going there are countless little jobs involved, too numerous and too small to list but they all become part of our daily process. For instance, one of those would be the preparation and the administration of medications. Some I prepare for the week while others I organize daily. Rita needs medication given to her nine times a day on a strict timed schedule. I commence at 7 am and give her the last dose at 10.15 pm. Anything from one tablet to six at any one time. Dealing with medications I have also found it helpful to have a cooperative pharmacist!

As earlier indicated, I find that each day is unpredictable. Numerous times I have said "Well, we won't do that again."We continually learn from each new experience. We go with the flow.

It may seem I treat Rita as a passive receiver of care, but Rita has a mind of her own and can share how she feels. For instance, we talk about her feelings related to finding herself in this untenable predicament. She is permanently in a place of helplessness and is unable to do very much for herself. This she finds very depressing. Parkinson's patients are prone to depression, and I can understand why. They have lost so much independence and Rita is no different. It has been essential for me to be aware of this and help to offset it if possible.

Rita has a strong faith and that helps considerably in overcoming the times of "feeling down."I try to bring encouragement by looking at, and sharing, the positive side of our lives. My reading to her also helps. We cannot change the circumstances but, in my caring, I attempt not to treat Rita as a patient but simply as my wife who is having to deal with this inconvenient illness. I maintain that we are facing the enemy of Parkinson's together. I am always on her side. I feel this attitude helps her feel she is not alone is dealing with this nasty on-going inca-pacity.

When we contemplate our life together, Rita, nor I, have never entertained the thought that life is unfair. What would that achieve? It certainly would not change anything. It would only create dissatisfaction and an atti-tude of self-pity. Life is as it is. We only have one life, so we make the most of it and enjoy it to the fullest extent possible. We take one day at a time because that is all we have. We try to live consciously in the now.

A Typical Day in the Life of the Murrays

6 am.	Wake Rita and take her to the bathroom and get her back to bed.
6.15 – 6.45	Shave and shower – (for myself that is)
6.45 – 7.00	Prepare medication for initial administration at 7 am
	Make some tea.
7 am	Get Rita up.
	Bathroom. Shower or wash. Underclothes on.
	Make up. Choose clothes for the day.
8 am	Care-Aid arrives to help with dressing
8.15. am	Help with hair and make-up.
8.30. am	Get Rita in the wheelchair and to the dining room for breakfast.
	Breakfast time medication

9.15. am   Finish breakfast and take a
            wheelchair walk around the
            building.

9.30. am   Get Rita back to the suite and
            bathroom for teeth-cleaning.

            Daily devotions

10 am   On two days a week Rita goes
            for 30-minute chair exercises.
            On Friday morning she goes to
            the hairdressers.

            On other days the mornings
            are free to listen to audio or
            watch TV. We also utilize this
            time for medical, dental, and
            other appointments.

11.45 am   Medication. Rita to the bath-
            room in preparation for lunch.

Noon   Rita into the wheelchair and go
            down for lunch followed by a
            walk outside ifweather permits.

1.30 -1.45 After lunch more medication
            and then get her set in her
            recliner chair for afternoon
            rest.

3.15 – 3.30 Wake Rita with afternoon
            refreshments.

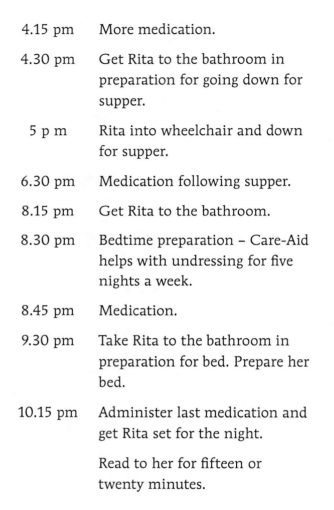

4.15 pm	More medication.
4.30 pm	Get Rita to the bathroom in preparation for going down for supper.
5 p m	Rita into wheelchair and down for supper.
6.30 pm	Medication following supper.
8.15 pm	Get Rita to the bathroom.
8.30 pm	Bedtime preparation – Care-Aid helps with undressing for five nights a week.
8.45 pm	Medication.
9.30 pm	Take Rita to the bathroom in preparation for bed. Prepare her bed.
10.15 pm	Administer last medication and get Rita set for the night.
	Read to her for fifteen or twenty minutes.

This is the skeleton of the day's activity. Obviously, there are many other things which fill in the gaps like laundry, washing a few dishes, cleaning up in the bathroom and many other daily jobs which happen in any normal household.

CHAPTER 3

What is Required of Me?

Every situation is different and has its own unique challenges. We have friends who are dealing with dementia and Alzheimer's, and they have their own set of distinctive problems and hurdles. I sense that their task is much greater than mine. With Parkinson's I think the slowness and inability of movement are the main obstacles to overcome, along with the problem of balance. Although there are many different symptoms which are termed Parkinsonian, most patients endure slowness and mobility issues. It can be the cause of much frustration in both the caregiver and those cared for.

With Rita everything happens astronomically slow. Anything that she can still do is painfully slow. It is like seeing life happen in slow motion. For instance, how long does it take to put on your glasses? Ten seconds? Maybe five? Maybe less? When I give Rita her glasses to put on, I know it will be almost a minute before they are in place, unless I help her.

We soon learned that time is not of the essence. I remember the day when Rita said, "Hurry is no longer in my vocabulary." She was right and we plan accordingly. There is little point in saying, "Hurry up," because that adds frustration to frustration. Besides, what's the rush? Where are we going? We tend not to get out and about very much now so why the hurry. In the overall scheme of things speed becomes less important.

If we do go out, then we try to allow ourselves adequate time for getting ready. I find to leave extra preparation time is the only solution or we adjust our thinking to accommodate delays. Something often goes wrong and at a time when you least need it to occur. One takes care not to allow frustration to bring on irritability, which is no help to anyone. As a caregiver I recognize my vulnerability to this when I am tired, exhausted, or just feel unwell. Regardless of how you feel, whatever is required must still be done. This adds pressure to the situation.

With Rita's constant slowness I avoid the temptation to jump in and do things because I know I can do them faster. I have found it necessary to resist that. I am here to help Rita be as independent as possible. I am taking the independence away if I keep jumping in to take over. I am sure it makes her feel worse if small things which she can do are snatched away. I have learned to be willing to allow, if necessary, things to take place at a snail's pace. Time is no longer important in these circumstances, but Rita's emotional health and her sense of well-being is. How much better for her to be praised for a small accomplishment than to be ready to go out of the house a couple of minutes earlier.

Sense of humour

One of the main things required of me is a sense of humour. Laughter is so important. It goes a long way to keeping things on an even keel. Nobody wants to be laughed at, but most enjoy being laughed with. We laugh at ourselves. We laugh at our situation. There are funny sides to many of the issues we deal with. I think the sentence, "If we didn't laugh, we would cry," probably has its rightful place here.

The times I have put her pants on back to front is hilarious. Bras on upside down, clothes on inside out and so on. Mishaps and mistakes happen but we make light of those things and laugh them away. Learning to cook and do the meals was another laughable occupation. I graduated from the initial boiled egg to something more substantial but not without mishaps on the way.

I cannot emphasize enough the benefits we have found in humour. We know that laughing lifts the spirits and enhances the immune system, therefore it can do nothing but help us in our caregiving situation. I even read a joke book to Rita once to give her a laugh. Laughter releases tension. It allows for joint acceptance of mistakes. It covers up awkwardness. A sense of humour will carry you through an otherwise tiresome day or help you to accept an otherwise upsetting occurrence. Laughter is certainly a good medicine.

One thing that has been a blessing for me is Rita's attitude. Her attitude to contracting Parkinson's has always been as positive as it can be having such an insidious disease. She has never said "Why me?" Only once has Rita ever asked the question "Why is life so difficult" which is not unreasonable considering her intolerable disposition. She has always done whatever has been required of her by the medical people and has been willing to follow advice.

Her attitude is even more astounding when you consider her current limitations in comparison with how active she was both physically and socially. Even after her diagnosis she continued leading a women's bible study group. Life would be very different, and more difficult for both of us, if Rita bemoaned her lot and was constantly unhappy. This is not so, and I am grateful. I am not saying she likes it, far from it, but her acceptance and resignation to the situation conveys to me a positive attitude.

Patience and understanding

Probably the main requirement of me in caregiving is patience and understanding, although the exercise of patience is probably the greatest requirement to do the job well. It takes patience to perform all the daily activities again and again and again. Getting clothes on and off someone who cannot help you is most difficult, even if the desire to cooperate is there. Even the mundane fastening of buttons and doing up zippers can be a problem.

I have always found however, that in most circumstances when there is a call to exercise patience, it is more beneficial to respond than react. Our tendency when we are irritated or frustrated, and that happens to the best of us, is that we are quick to react instead of a thoughtful and calculated response. I know time is not always on our side in particular situations but to react harshly is to regret it later and upsetting to both.

When anyone is incapacitated or ill, bathroom accidents happen when you least expect it. An unexpected change of clothes is not uncommon and calls for patience and understanding. Some tasks are unwelcome, irksome, unpleasant, and difficult. Then taking care of personal issues can be a delicate and sensitive task. I think I have learned more about women's personal hygiene and care than I ever needed to know.

Sensitivity is also required when in public. Consider restaurants for instance. I try to assist Rita as unobtrusively as possible, not making a show of it. Often her food needs to be cut up which is better done with the plate in front of me, instead of her. It is natural that incapacities bring on self-consciousness and even embarrassment. In my public caring, I try to minimize and alleviate that as much as possible.

While we are talking about restaurants let me share with you probably the biggest disservice, we have found in that setting. There is in the minds of many the equation that to be physically incapacitated means a lack of mental ability. Because Rita has mobility problems it is assumed that her mental capabilities are equally deficient. Consequently, I get the third person treatment and am asked "What would she want?" or "What about her?" This is galling as Rita is quite capable of choosing and ordering for herself. I have been known to give a simple but gentle answer. "Her name is Rita, and she is quite competent to make her own decisions, ask her."Sadly, this link between physical and mental incapacities is not uncommon. Other friends have indicated they have received similar treatment. It's unfortunate but it happens.

Obviously, our situation is not without its frustration and irritations – we are human after all! However, I have found a way to avoid frustration turning into annoyance. It is simply to remind myself that Rita has not chosen to be like this. She would prefer to be otherwise. She would prefer to be independent as she once was. She would love to be as active as others are around her. She did nothing to bring on this illness. Her limitations are not self-imposed. She cannot help moving so slowly. It is not her fault that she takes so long to sit down or is slow in taking her medicine. It is natural for her to be anxious about the potentiality of falling and hold tightly on the various surfaces and bury her fingernails into my hands for security.

It's not her fault

By remembering that it is not her fault, I immediately am on her side and look at life from her point of view. You recognize all the restrictions she faces and get the sense that, inwardly she must feel so frustrated and maybe justifiably annoyed at her situation, although she never shows it. If Rita's deterioration is hard for me to see and accept, it must be even harder and most depressing for her. While I keep these thoughts of her helplessness in mind, it enhances in me patience and understanding.

Another aspect of Rita's care which is very important to me is, how she looks. Rita has always taken pride in her appearance, and I see no reason why it should not continue, even if she must be presented to the world in a wheelchair. So, before we go out, or even just to the dining room, I ensure that her hair has been combed, her clothes match and are clean, so she feels happy about the way she looks. Not for one moment do I want her to feel any embarrassment about her appearance.

There is a common problem which affects people confined to a wheelchair or who carry the appearance of their incapacity. It is this. They are often ignored in conversations. I have found the need to take proactive steps in situations where Rita feels redundant or feels left out in discussions. For instance, when we visit the doctor or see a specialist, they can so easily, but unintentionally, ignore Rita and ask me the questions relating to her health. I know it is difficult for Rita to answer quickly because of the Parkinson's, but she does have the answers and she should be heard. It is important for her to express how she sees her situation and how she feels inwardly about the progression of the disease. It is her body which is being discussed so I attempt to keep Rita involved in the conversation and the discussions with the medical professionals. This, I believe, is important for her sense of being accepted for who she is and being treated as an intelligent person who is quite capable of contributing to the evaluation.However, this applies not just during medical appointments. The same thing can occur with anyone with whom we talk. It is easy for people to start talking only to me. This, I try to avoid.

Caregiving and self-sacrifice inevitably go together like apple pie and ice cream. Yet the thought is worse than its reality. One realizes early on that the person one is caring for must come first, well, that is how I think of Rita. However much I might like to be doing something else, my first responsibility is to care for Rita, and I think it is good she knows that. I suppose this is what could be classed as self-sacrifice although I don't think of it that way. I believe if you are motivated by love then the sacrifice aspect fades away. Yes, it is still hard work, and it does not take away the times of exhaustion, but the tasks are not accompanied by any feelings of resentment. It becomes a pleasure to be available.

So, what is required of me to deal with Rita's condition and situation? Mostly an understanding heart and of course, physical strength. I always keep in my mind that Rita is Rita and not Parkinson's or PSP. She is not the disease but is grossly affected by the illness. I am always able to see the real Rita behind the symptoms. In the context of spousal care, I will always say that nothing can take the place of love. I am not talking about a sense of pity or sympathy but loving the person for who they are. I know that Rita needs to know and experience that love daily. She needs to know that whatever occurs I will be there to love her through it.

I know there are some wonderful Care-aid workers, and some excellent staff in care homes, who are kindness

personified and do a superb job, but there is a deeper relationship in spousal care when love is the basis. Nothing
can replace the love between spouses, or between children and parents. Love overrides the rough spots and
overcomes many obstacles.

CHAPTER 4

Is There a Limit?

All illnesses bring limitations and Parkinson's is no exception. Activities which were once a regular part of life are curtailed or even discontinued. Limitations hit you at different levels and in different ways. As physical movement has become more difficult for Rita, so it has brought a limitation to our daily activities together. Our program has had to be adjusted. We have learned to accept that which we cannot change. It is easier to go with the flow, change arrangements and implement new ones. But in considering this word limit, there is a more personal application which is very real and is a big issue with all caregivers.

Probably the two biggest limitations which caregivers face are, at what stage do I reach my limit physically and at what stage do I look to get help. We will look at the question of personal limit in this chapter and consider the question of help in the next. The serious aspect about the personal physical limit is this; if I do not recognize my physical limit then I could well move into a situation where my care for Rita becomes inadequate, and maybe unsafe.

In a nutshell, yes there is a limit, but the problem is knowing where that limit is and then being willing to acknowledge it. There obviously is a limit to one's strength and ability to care. However, to determine the point in time when the caring process is more difficult than one can manage, is hard to know. I think, or like to think, that I will always have endless energy and that my strength will go on for years. My son periodically reminds me that I get older by the month and my strength inevitably declines with the passing of time. The real danger arises when I fail to recognize my inability to care properly for Rita. That puts her at risk.

In 2010, two years after Rita was diagnosed with Parkinson's, we made a big decision to move 3000 miles from Ontario, in central Canada, to British Columbia on the west coast of Canada. This was encouraged by family, and it proved to be a wise move. Although we had no idea of how soon we might need help, we knew it would happen one day. As expected, it has happened since we arrived here, and we did require help. I have had several bouts of vertigo and two emergency visits to the hospital in that time and we needed help to care for Rita.

Then in 2015 we moved into a Retirement Community which has a resident nurse and Care-aid workers. We did that in the event we might need help on a daily basis as well as in an emergency situation. In addition, we knew that the Retirement Community had a full-care floor which Rita may need one day.

No more travel

Rita says that Parkinson's has stolen parts of our life and she is right. It has robbed us of opportunities to travel, of spending more time with family and the blessings of social interaction with church friends. But that is all negative and we try not to dwell on the downside of life.

Travel is probably the biggest practical limitation. Whether by plane or perhaps even by car, it is no longer easy although a car would be easier than the plane. Long-distance travel is now virtually a non-starter. Vacations are a thing of the past. If a trip had to be made for family reasons, then I am sure we would do it, but to deliberately put ourselves into such a position does not make sense. It would be somewhat inconvenient for me, but very difficult and extremely stressful for Rita. Before we made any decision about travel, I think we would question its advisability and examine the ultimate benefit.

It is sad to realize that places to which we have been will not be visited again. This is where memories are important – to remember what we did and where we went, what we saw and whose company we enjoyed. We may not be able to plan vacations anymore, but I guess every day we are retired is a vacation day!

Life changes constantly for every one of us, but more so in the caregiving situation. Hopes, dreams, aspirations, expectations all change as the disease progresses. Plans are made, changed, or adapted according to feasibility. Sadly, over the years even connections with friends have lessened. It is so nice when you hear from a friend who wants to drop by. Facebook has been a positive vehicle in that respect and allowed us to keep in touch with many friends who would otherwise have been lost through lack of physical connection. Emails also have been invaluable.

Regrettably, determined by our limitations, the living room has virtually become our world. Unfortunately, you get to the stage when you find going out is no longer as convenient as it once was. As indicated earlier our trips out are dictated by necessity, mostly doctors, dentists, or other medical appointments – not very exciting!

To avoid the sense of entrapment indoors, we attempt to enjoy whatever it is we do inside. We try not to have the television on without reason although it is good company when you need it. We choose our programs and watch what we enjoy. We are avid armchair sports fans enjoying tennis, soccer, rugby, and snooker, to name some of the sports we follow. We may not be there in person, but we are there in spirit and delight in the wins of those we support.

Physical limitations

Looking at my own personal limitations, I admit to finding them most difficult to accept. For some time, these have been my on-going thoughts, "I am the husband. Husbands are supposed to care for their wives and take care of all issues that need putting right. I am the man of the house; I should be strong and invincible." However, through the years of caring, I have come to realize that this is not always the case. I have discovered, surprisingly, that I am human and not superman, as I might wish. I have learned that I get tired and exhausted. In my 80 odd years of life, I have never had to sleep in the daytime but am now finding I am falling asleep while watching television, which is annoying if it is soccer. Sometimes I feel like Scrooge in *A Christmas Carol* when he says "I am not the man I was" although the application might not be the same, the words do apply. As the years have progressed, I have also found it strange that the wheelchair gets heavier each time I lift it in and out of the car.

There are days that I feel on top of the world and think I can do this job forever. There are also days when

I wonder if I can see the month out. A point of real concern was when I woke up one morning to realize that anything and everything that is to be done has to be done by me, and to realize that it was not just for that day, but from there on in, every day! That thought was daunting and disturbing.

What I find even more disturbing now is when I wake up already feeling exhausted before the day starts. It is at those times when you feel weak and vulnerable. However, you continue to find the strength to swing your legs out of bed - although I am not sure about the swinging part – and approach another day of caring. The realization hits you that this is your life and things are not going to change, except perhaps get busier and perhaps more difficult. Mentally you accept it and press on.

Some days life appears to be harder for Rita, both physically and mentally, which makes the day harder for me. On those days she requires greater physical help. At times I think optimistically that I see improvements in her condition only to realize that they are temporary in nature. Sadly, we cannot turn the clock back and you come to accept that things will not return to former days or how things once were. It is hard to accept that Rita will not again be how she once was. Most people would remember her as active, quick witted, having a pleasant disposition and good company. Not that these personality aspects have disappeared, but her body no longer allows her to be active. She is still quick-witted even if the response time has been slowed down by Parkinson's. She is still good company in a one-to-one setting. However, as her voice has become weaker, crowds are no longer her cup of tea.

I am well aware of various studies on the health and well-being of caregivers. It is estimated that a third of caregivers see a drastic decline in health as well as age prematurely and that 60% of caregivers die before the person for whom they are caring. This is not something one wants to hear or read about but it is reality. However, there are caregivers who appear to be able to adapt to the task, handle it well and even find themselves blessed by the experience. I would like to be one of those people. The reality is, most caregivers are subject to a lack of sleep and unfortunately sleep deprivation has an adverse effect upon the immune system, which does not bode well for catching infections which may be going around. It can also bring on anxiety and depression along with a decline in a sense of well-being.

Stress and guilt

Chronic stress can also hit the immune system hard. With caregiving, stress cannot be eliminated but I try to avoid it. Obviously, I do not wish to burn out and crash because then I would be no good to myself or Rita. One learns to say and appreciate the prayer that Reinhold Niebuhr left for us, "God grant me the serenity to accept the things that I cannot change, the courage to change the things I can and the wisdom to know the difference."

We hear again and again from many well-meaning people and medical professionals, "Take care of yourself!"Our doctor said those words and added, "If you are not around, who will care for Rita?" The big question in the mind is "How do you do that?"The need to do it is well understood but to work out the details of time away, respire care and time for self, is a bigger problem than many might imagine. One cannot just walk away.

Before the pandemic restrictions I had a person come in once a week for 90 minutes so I could go out, have a coffee, and enjoy my book for an hour. The pandemic changed all that and it has been well over eighteen months since I have been able to get that kind of break. Since those days Rita's voice has become weaker and she finds conversations with visitors in person, and on the telephone, very difficult. Also, with her constant tiredness she finds the effort of entertaining quite exhausting.

I also carry a sense of guilt for even wanting to be away from Rita for any length of time. There is no basis for that. That is just a personal sense of loyalty to my wife. However, I know taking breaks is a must, otherwise the stress of a 24/7 care schedule will come back to bite me. Exercise helps but that too calls for time and discipline.

Right now, the pandemic restrictions are beginning to ease and hopefully soon there will be more accommodation to having visitors and allow for organizing specific breaks for respite.

I know I have failed in organizing respite. Not only would it be beneficial for me, but it would also help Rita get used to other people providing the care. This is a big issue. Rita is a private person and finds it so difficult when it comes to others being involved in her personal care. I respect that and I know it is not uncommon. Many of those cared for get used to the caregiver they have and are reluctant to have other people involved. Knowing that sensitivity in Rita, it is easy for me to go along with that sentiment and think that I should be the one to always do the caring. Even worse is for me to think I am the only one who can care for her, which, of course, is not true. These are all self-limiting thoughts and are not helpful to Rita or me.

So where am I with considering a limit? I like to think there is no reason why we could not go on for years and I hope we do, however, that may be somewhat unrealistic. Obviously, we need to be prepared for the day when it is no longer possible. If I am honest, I am probably in a state of limbo, knowing that a limit will be reached at some point, but I like to think it is not yet.

As has happened with many people, there is the temptation to push beyond the limit, but I do not wish for a moment to be a dead hero – that is no good to anyone! I am trusting it will become clear to me when that limit is reached. In fact, I am hoping that we both will know when the limit is reached and that we both will be accepting of the change it inevitably will bring. I am aware of the danger in waiting too long. I certainly don't want to wait until I hit the brick wall because that would not be helpful. Yet, I also do not want to quit while I have the strength to keep going.

My back, shoulders, arms, and fingers may hurt from the physical aspect of caring over these past years, but I am pleased with the fact that I can still do what I need to do in my daily caring for Rita, so for now, I can and will keep going.

CHAPTER 5

When Should I Get Help?

Getting help does not present such a dilemma as trying to recognize where my physical limit is. I can more quickly recognize the need for help and am willing to admit it. Admitting your limit is a much bigger decision as its implications are far reaching and serious. It is much easier to accept physical help than to say I have reached my limit and can go no further.

It has taken a while, but now I try not to go beyond what I can reasonably carry out. If something is too much to handle, then I have become willing to admit it. It was hard initially but I am no longer afraid to ask for help, both inside and outside the family. This I have found pleasantly reassuring because when I have approached someone for help, I have been surprised just how quick, ready, and willing they are to help. I refer mostly to people running errands for us. Actual help in physically caring for Rita is a different scenario and presents greater difficulties.

Every caregiver needs help, and I am no exception. I understand that the ideal recommended scenario is to gather a "care" team around you, which sounds easier than it is. Some situations encompassing serious medical issues even call for having a medically qualified person available for consultation. My situation does not call for that. For my care team it has been family and friends although, as well, we are blessed with a wonderful husband and wife team for our regular doctors. They have shown so much genuine concern in caring for Rita.

Our family has given incredible support in a variety of ways during these years of caregiving, especially doing a superb job of shopping for us during the pandemic. Several friends from church have also been involved in regular errand running for us, taking shirts to the cleaners, books to the post office and buying items from the supermarket. We are indebted to all those who have stepped up to the plate to help us in that capacity.

Misguided thinking

I am sure you have already sensed that I don't exactly have it all together in some areas of this caregiving job and the following will just confirm it. There are internal struggles which I know should not be there. When I think about getting help, I find that I have the erroneous thinking that I am showing weakness or falling down on my responsibility. I am trying hard to learn that I am not a failure if I ask for help. Also, that it is not "heartless" to want a break, especially for health reasons. Feeling guilty about needing a respite or even entertaining that idea is very real for me. In my mind it presents itself as though I want, or am willing, to abandon Rita, Obviously, that is far from the truth. It hinges back to my misguided thinking that as a man, and as the husband, I should be able to handle everything and deal with the fatigue. I have this sense that I am thinking more about myself than Rita. I know I need to change my thinking and get a better perspective on the situation. Unfortunately, what I am succumbing to is not uncommon, it is a classic case of caregiver guilt, the guilt of abandonment – even when it really does not exist.

As a caregiver I know I need support from other people, both mentally and physically. Both are equally important. I read this somewhere and understand the truth of this principle that "we fail to ask for help to our own peril."

However, at what stage in caregiving do you start looking for help? Although no one task could be classified as being too big or too hard, life as a caregiver is made up of a myriad of regular tasks. When you combine them altogether you recognize the danger that eventually one small task might prove to be the inevitable straw which breaks the camel's back. I refer of course to the proverbial brick wall. I am often reminded of the phrase "I can do anything, but I can't do everything."

I must admit that my intelligence—yes, I do have some--reminds me that not to get appropriate help at the proper time will eventually take its toll on my physical and emotional health. However, unless it is something significant like a heart attack, it is not easy to recognize a decline in your own health. Others see what we cannot see in ourselves. A friend told me that he had no idea of how far down the hill his health had gone until he stopped his 24/7 care for his wife. Nobody wants to burn-out.

A husband knows what his wife likes and dislikes. He knows what upsets her. He senses her feelings in different circumstances. He knows when she needs to rest and when she wants to be quiet and relax. He also knows when she is troubled and disturbed inwardly without verbally expressing anything. This alone should qualify us as good caregivers. I know these things about Rita, but because I have this knowledge, it does not mean that I am the only person who can give her proper care. There is no reason why others cannot learn the same things and offer her the same care. It is a fallacy for me to think otherwise, but sometimes hard to shake from the mind.

These are some of the issues with which I struggle mentally.

What is respite?

I have discovered that respite means different things to different people. To some it simply means a change, a break, doing something other than the caring responsibilities. It certainly means getting your mind onto something else, maybe reading, playing a sport, or going to a concert. It may mean a change of venue to enjoy an evening of quietness and rejuvenation. I find writing to be a diversion and a helpful change from regular caregiving activity but that is not respite. I think it goes deeper than that. For me respite means that I can walk away and leave Rita confidently in the care of someone else. If I read or write in the same location as my wife, then I continue to be responsible for her. However, if I feel that someone else is responsible – even for an hour or so – that to me is respite.

Help comes for the caregiver in different forms. For some long time before the pandemic, I was able to meet with a friend for coffee while Rita rested. He would visit here in the building. We enjoyed the time together, and it was a support to me. Sometimes a caregiver just simply needs a cup of coffee and an understanding ear. That will make the day. The importance of support from friends is crucial. To receive a phone call, text message or email gives an incredible boost for the day. It provides strength. It tells you that you are not forgotten, and that people care for you.

As I have mentioned some of our closest friends are having to deal with dementia which is extremely difficult to handle. One of the blessings we enjoy is that, although Rita is incapacitated physically, she has no cognitive problems, which is a huge positive factor when communication is normal. Rita is well up on world events and current affairs. We watch the news together, discuss situations in the news and as I have said previously, we are armchair sport fans, so time spent together is often enjoyed that way. Doing things together is relaxing and at the same time I am there if needed. Just being together is of utmost importance. It is one more aspect of making the most of the time we have together.

It is mentally healthy and important for caregivers to have other side interests and mine has been writing. While Rita rests for 90 minutes each afternoon and occasionally when she is watching a television program in which I have no interest, I can turn to reading or writing. This book is the fifth book I have written since Rita contracted Parkinson's.

It was about two years ago when I began to recognize that I needed help. That would have been eleven years after Rita's diagnosis, so I started getting help with dressing and undressing her during the week while I continued that task on the weekends. We have recently increased the morning help to seven days a week. However, I do recognize that more help is going to be needed and maybe sooner than later. It makes sense that the more help I can get, the longer we stay together.

So, to answer the question posed at the beginning of the chapter, when should I get help? Rather than waiting until we know our strength is waning, it is wise to be proactive and get things in motion sooner rather than later. When is the right time? The answer is always, just before we need it. The problem is, who knows when that is?

CHAPTER 6

Is There a Spiritual Side to This?

For me, there is a spiritual side to life and thus a spiritual aspect to caregiving. However, let me be quick to point out that there are hundreds of thousands of people doing an admirable job as caregivers who would not profess to have a faith or perhaps any religious connection. I only speak from my own perspective and am not, in any way, suggesting that a faith is a prerequisite to adequately perform the task of caregiving. However, if I did not mention it, I would not be giving you an honest or balanced picture of our life.

As Christians our faith is important to us. The Church is important. Christian friends are important. In fact, their importance has become even more accentuated as I operate in an active caregiving role. Before the pandemic hit in 2020, we made the effort to be in church each Sunday morning. It was not without its struggles. Even getting up at six in the morning, as usual, we were still hard-pressed to be prepared to leave at 9.30 am. Remember, I have two people to get ready to leave the apartment. We normally made it on time but eventually, I removed the time constraints from my mind and decided that to get to church was an achievement, and to get there on time was a bonus. We usually managed the bonus!

Our personal faith influences our attitudes and outlook on life and has been a permanent benefit to us as we find strength and grace from our faith in God. It helps us through the days when things go wrong and when the situation appears most difficult. Those are the days we need God-given patience and understanding. We pray together and find consolation in doing so as we present to God issues that we might be facing at that moment as well as what might be around the corner for us. We feel the assurance that God knows and cares. There are times when the best action is to step back, take your hands off and let God take over and work things out according to his purpose.

The power of prayer

Most conversations are normally two-sided and as prayer is a conversation with God, it is no different. From prayer we derive comfort, wisdom, strength, discernment, and understanding. Without us telling him, God knows how we feel. He knows the difficulties we might be going through and the obstacles we face. He also knows our heart and understands our wishes and desires. It is no big job for him to give us the strength to go through the difficult days and deal with problems which inevitably arise in all caregiving scenarios. I believe God can take care of any situation we might find ourselves in. We have learned to trust him.

We also receive comfort when we hear that, others are praying for us. It provides us with encouragement which is never amiss in caregiving. I honestly believe we are blessed when others pray. It is one more thing which tells us that people care and are standing with us in the daily battle.

Reading the Bible and praying together brings us closer to God. God brings hope and comfort. It gives us a sense of confidence and spiritual security. God is never far away. He has promised to never leave us or forsake us, and we have learned in life that God keeps his promises. The Bible states "The Lord is close to the brokenhearted and saves those who are crushed in spirit." (Psalm 34:18.) Hence, we are not alone, however much we feel like it sometimes. Yet in our times of heartache, sadness, and disappointments he is there upholding us without our knowledge or understanding. He is there also in the good times when we feel upbeat because things are going well. It is at those times that we need to remember to be grateful and offer our thanksgiving.

Most people have read the story of "Footprints in the sand." I feel it has a particular application for caregivers so let me remind you of it here. A man dreamt that he was walking on the beach with the Lord. At the same time scenes from his life were flashing across the sky. He also noticed there were two sets of footprints in the sand except when he was at the lowest and saddest point in his life. Not understanding this, he asked the Lord why it was that at these particular times when he needed him most, he had seemingly left him. The Lord replied "My precious child. I love you and would never leave you. During your times of trial and suffering, when you see only one set of footprints, it was then that I carried you."Caregiving for some people can be a very lonely job. How nice to know that at our lowest point the Lord will carry us through.

A Christian is a follower of Jesus, which means that Jesus is the teacher, and I am the student. As a student I must learn what Jesus teaches and how it applies to my everyday life. Consequently, I need to learn how his teaching applies to the way I care for Rita. St Paul actually encourages us to think like Christ, to adopt the mind of Christ. To do so we need to know him, his characteristics, his attitude, and his very spirit. As I know that Jesus would bring love, compassion, and comfort into any situation. That is my guide in caregiving.

I am reminded of the example of Jesus in washing his disciple's feet. Can you imagine. They had been walking in sandals on dry dusty roads and here was, not just a Rabbi but, the very Son of God, washing their dirty feet. What a supreme example of humility and love. If Jesus could do that and I am following his example, then there is nothing that I should not be willing to do for Rita.

There is a popular phrase which some consider to be trite, but I think it applies here. The phrase is "What would Jesus do?"It is a question that we are encouraged to answer when we are faced with bewildering situations. In performing the multiple tasks before me as a caregiver I find it helpful to have this phrase within my mind. It is especially applicable in the exercise of patience over frustration and a calm response as opposed to an irritated reaction to any given situation.

It also helps avoid the temptation of raising one's voice. I have been known to occasionally increase the volume when trying to emphasize a point or reacting to a potentially dangerous situation. Rita interprets it as shouting and comes back with "Don't shout at me!"Even when I am just trying to emphasize the urgency, it can come across as shouting which is unhelpful at any time.

As Christians I believe we reflect God's love in caregiving. As we do things in love the difficult tasks do not necessarily get easier but sometimes, they feel easier to handle and allow us to embrace tasks which otherwise we might not relish.

To illustrate the kind of love which fits somewhat into the scenario of caring is a biblical passage which is often read at wedding ceremonies. It describes love in its perfection. Let me quote "Love is patient, love is kind. It does not envy, it does not boast, it is not proud. It is not rude, it is not self-seeking, it is not easily angered, it keeps no record of wrongs. Love does not delight in evil but rejoices with the truth. It always protects, always trusts, always hopes, always perseveres." (I Cor. 13:4-7) To me this passage of Scripture is a constant reminder to always be patient and kind, not easily becoming angry, always protecting Rita, offering her constant hope and persevere in our situation regardless of what we face together.

Some suggest there is a deeper spiritual application for the Christian in caregiving. It is thought that being called to such a task helps to transform the caregiver more into the image of Christ. What does that mean? I understand it to mean that the caregiver's life should display some of the characteristics of Christ. When I think of my every-day activity, it is not difficult to see how some of those characteristics are needed to do the job. Think about love, patience, gentleness, meekness – all full within the image and character of Christ. What a privilege to know that all the obstacles we face, the things that go wrong, the everyday mundane duties, are all teaching me to be more like Christ. Putting that into context makes the task even more a privilege than I had previously thought.

Our faith is tested

Our faith allows us to face life's challenges and brings confidence and assurance that all will be well. Not that everything is put right but as Christians we know that God is aware of our situation, he loves and cares for both of us. We are assured he will take care and work things out according to his purpose and with our interest in mind. We certainly do not understand everything in life, but this is where our faith is tested and is ultimately rewarded. In the caregiving role our faith is certainly tested.

Although our faith may be challenged by circum-stances, if we are assured that God knows and cares, our faith becomes stronger and creates the support and undergirding that we need at that moment. Just as the caregiver brings hope and security to those cared for, so God brings hope and confidence to caregivers. He sees us through the bad patches, the days when exhaustion is the norm. I like the quotation by John Dunlop in his book *Finding Grace in the Face of Dementia* where he says, "God is the caregiver's caregiver." I believe that is true in principle and in practice. People will ask, "How do you cope?" My answer is always "With God's help!"

There are days when you think "I cannot do this alone." It is on such days when I believe God steps in to provide me with the strength I need for that day. There is a strength which even surprises me, not physical but spiritual. I believe it helps me face the difficulties and disappointments of everyday caregiving. It does not change the situation or make things any less painful, but it does seem to provide the strength to overcome and rise above an unenviable situation.

Believing that we are in God's hands gives confidence and consolation that whatever is in the present and whatever lies before us will be His concern as well. From this comes an inner peace and inexplicable strength. None of us know what the future holds but the Christian knows who holds the future. Having the assurance that God is in control and has our interest at heart is very comforting as we face an uncertain future. Because we have no control over the situation or the disease, we have no alternative but to hand things over to God and trust implicitly in Him.

Another important aspect in caregiving is having an attitude of gratefulness. I try to always have a grateful heart. Gratefulness lifts the spirit. It helps me see the positive side of issues. It reminds me that things could always be worse. Regardless of our circumstances there is always something for which to be grateful for in life.

As I have indicated before, I believe God has entrusted me with caring for Rita, so it is a privilege to do so. I want to be able to stand before God one day and say, "I cared for Rita the very best way I possibly could."I see my role as Rita's caregiver as a call from God. He knew Rita would need care and chose me to give it to her. However, the process is beneficial to me as well because, as indicated earlier, I believe it moulds and changes my character to be more Christ-like, which is the very purpose of being a Christian.

I like to think that I serve God as I serve my wife. I seek to honour God as I care for Rita. I believe God uses our hands, arms, and bodies to do his will and be a blessing to others. I think this is particularly applicable in the caregiving role. I may feel inadequate for the job and even be inadequate, but I believe God gives me daily strength and makes me strong enough for the task he has called me to do. I honestly believe without God's help I would have been finished years ago!

CHAPTER 7

What About Tomorrow?

Anyone suffering from a progressive disease inevitably contemplates, with some trepidation, what the future may hold. We are no different. With Rita as victim of the disease and myself as the caregiver, we have no idea of what tomorrow may hold. Yes, it is true, we have a faith and that gives us confidence that ultimately all will be well, but we are still human and passing through various stages of life bring with them various emotions. Consequently, thoughts of uncertainty and not knowing exactly what lies ahead elicits an element of concern. I naturally try, but it is hard to totally eliminate that kind of concern, especially for Rita. We talk about all possibilities regarding the future. I have always tried to be positive about life and am no different in this scenario.

It is one thing to talk about a plan and even make one, but plans are never fool proof. Hopefully having a potential plan takes away some concern regarding the unknown. However, you can only plan so much. Not all contingencies can be covered. Things can change very quickly – a sudden fall or an unexpected illness for either of us and the future becomes very cloudy. We could immediately be thrust into an unplanned and maybe unwanted change – perhaps forever.

Looking squarely at the future is difficult. There is no magic pill that makes all the downside of our situation go away and cause everything in the garden to be lovely. I also realize the task will get no easier than it is today, which is not a pleasant prospect to contemplate. The demands will grow, and the responsibilities will grow. Individual routine activities will become more difficult. As I have indicated in a previous chapter, the greater difficulty will be recognizing when we have come to the end of the road. Nobody wants that day to arrive. It is very disturbing to even think about it. How can one ever mentally prepare for separation?

Naturally neither of us want to be separated ever. At this moment the very idea of separation is abhorrent to both of us. However, we do recognize that the day will come when Rita needs more care than I can give her. How we would like to delay the arrival of that day. To both of us, obtaining more help here in our home is more desirable than having Rita away elsewhere. Just now she needs me, and I need her to be here. My heart says that I want to be there caring for her to the absolute end.

Even knowing how infantile these questions may sound, my mind continually wrestles with issues about separation such as, how can others care for Rita as I do, without knowing her as I do? How would they know how to take care of her in the bathroom? Who will put toothpaste on her brush? Who will be there at mealtimes to cut up her food and help her eat? Who will wipe her mouth and ensure that her face is clean? Who will remember to give her medications on time, nine times a day? Who? Who? Who? The questions go on.

I find it emotionally disturbing to consider that Rita may need to go into full care simply because I can no longer provide the extent of care she needs. That gives me the sense of being the cause for her being there, although deep down, I know that is not true. It certainly creates a feeling of inadequacy on my part. I assume the best way to handle it is to consider it like hospitalization. If Rita needed hospital care, then that would seem to be more readily acceptable to me.

Like others in our situation, we live with a certain level of concern about the future. I purposely use the word concern, as opposed to fear and trepidation. Those words create for me the sense of expecting something nasty to suddenly come upon us. Something will happen eventually but hopefully it will not be nasty. When you have a concern, you do all you can to avoid the consequences or attempt to alleviate it. For instance, we live with the potentiality of Rita falling and which is one of our main concerns, so we now take every possible precaution to avoid any fall – although it still happens but perhaps less so than it might.

Here is an interesting question. If this was to be your last day together with your spouse, how would you want to remember it? I don't think of this constantly but as I care for Rita, I do have in the back of my mind that any day could be our last together. I do not think that in a morbid way, or in a pessimistic way, but just my attempt at being realistic. It gives me cause to make the day as pleasant as possible for both of us.

I remember listening to a television interview with a Japanese man who lost his wife and daughter in the Japanese tsunami. He indicated that they had had a terrible row before he went to work that morning. The tsunami came and swept away his wife and daughter. The last memory he had was the harsh words between them. That memory has been devastating to him ever since.

I don't expect a tsunami, but I do realize that a major change could come upon us quite unexpectedly. Hopefully we are living in a way that each of us enjoys and neither of us will have regrets if such a change suddenly occurs. This is another reason for us to appreciate and enjoy each other while we have the opportunity.

I am reminded of Joan Didion's book *The Year of Magical Thinking*. In it she aptly relates her feelings after losing her husband who collapsed at their dinner table. In her poignant description of the moment, she opens her book with the words, "Life changes fast. Life changes in the instant. You sit down to dinner and life as you know it ends."Such powerful and relevant words. As a caregiver such sentiment is never far from the mind.

The question of dying

Do we talk about dying? Yes, we talk about dying. Not a lot, but it does come up in conversation. It is not a usual topic over breakfast, but we have given it due consideration. As death is something which will happen to us all, it makes sense to talk about it, especially when you have illness thrown into the mix. Neither of us relish the thought that one day we will be separated by death. How comforting it is for the Christian to know that we are promised eternal life after this one and we'll meet again in that place Jesus said he was going to prepare.

Naturally there is always an element of concern and perhaps fear of what might be involved when we pass away. Rita is so reliant upon my being around it is obvious that she would immediately need full care. As Christians we live with the assurance of God's love and care and know that he is in control, however, we cannot but help look at how things might play out in the natural, even if our hearts know that truth.

The harsh reality is that if I die first then obviously there is no one to care for Rita. She would come under that care of the local health authority. This would also apply if I suffered a long-term illness. I am told Rita would first be taken into hospital and then because she would not be there to require medical treatment, she would subsequently be sent to a long-term care facility. If Rita dies first then, although not easier for me emotionally, it would be easier in that I would just need to find suitable accommodation.

We have also talked about making funeral arrangements while we are living, which helps the family once death occurs. I find it essential when thinking about the future that other members of our family know our thinking, our long term wishes and all the details about personal finances and know where to find the appropriate papers. I am trying to avoid unnecessary surprises along the way.

It is a known fact that, all of us think more about the events of yesterday and the future than we do of the present day. So, like others we too have tomorrow on the mind. But talking about tomorrow and the future is probably more significant in a caregiving situation as any major change affects the whole scenario. Being realistic we know we are in the evening of our lives, regardless of our physical conditions.

Death is inevitable, but we all naturally like to hold on to life, so I think most of us tend to divert our attention on to something else. We know it happens to others, but we also know deep down it will happen to us. So, however difficult, we need to be prepared for that day if we ever can be. I like the following quotation made by Chaplain William Sloane Coffin Jr. "The art of living is to die young, as late as possible."

Yesterday has gone, we have no idea what tomorrow may bring, which is probably a very good thing. We only have today. So, we try to appreciate it while we can.

While thinking about the topic of dying, I wrote a poem for Rita and would like to share it with you. I heard a poem along similar lines and have used the first line of that poem and added my own words from there. Here it is. You will see I am not much of a poet, in fact I know nothing about writing poetry, but the words carry some sentiment.

My Rita

If you go first and I remain.
I'll remember the joy and not the pain.
I'll remember the laughter and not the tears.
And all the special moments, down the years.

If you go first and I remain
I'll remember the sun and not the rain
I'll forget the struggles and remember the gain.
Living on little, enjoying the life
Thinking of victories and not the strife.

If you go first and I remain
I'll remember your love, your smile, your gentle spirit
Your thoughtful attitude and all that went with it.
The pleasant hours of thoughtful contemplation
Along with quiet moments of meditation.

If you go first and I remain
Watch for me, for the days will be few
When I will follow and again be with you.
Listen for me, I will be calling your name.
Look for me because I will be doing the same.
Looking for you, my dear Rita, just looking for you!

CHAPTER 8

Love Finds a Way!

In the busyness of everyday caring, it is easy to overlook physical affection. We may love our spouses, parents, or children immensely, but they need to be aware of it. I remember Rita saying one day not that long ago, "Can I have a hug?" It was then that I realized she needed a physical affectionate touch rather the constant manhandling of putting her in and out of her chair or wheelchair. Because the handling and touching is constant, I found I had forgotten that affection was more than just caring.

Because Rita's balance is virtually non-existent, I spend much time just holding her up. It is easy to be close, arms around her, but that is not a hug. I find that the hug must be a definitive action. It must be a real hug and the good thing is, it is never out of place. Since Rita mentioned it, I have tried to remember, not always so well. There are other ways by which we can convey love physically, an affectionate pat, a stroke, a touch, a gentle caress, or an appropriate word. All these go a long way to send the message of love. They may be little things, but they carry with them the words "I love you!" I also verbally assure Rita of my love every night before she sleeps.

A marriage commitment

When I first started out in this caregiving role it obviously wasn't an overnight occurrence. It crept up on me because it was just the natural process of life and part of our marriage relationship. However, as time has gone on it has become something very different. Initially it probably started out fulfilling a duty and responsibility, but my thinking changed and adapted to the role as love began to surround, and even motivate, the duties. I found that even when tired, there was still a certain joy in caring for Rita. I know I have mentioned this already, but I honestly believe that God entrusted me with this special task and therefore I consider it a privilege to care for the one I love.

For a long time, I have been sensitive to the fact that even in my mind, Rita could have become diminished to being just a patient who needs care, but she is not, she is my wife. She is also a mother, grandmother, and great-grandmother. Alongside that, in considering who I am and my role, it could be that I am just a caregiver, but I am not. I am first and foremost Rita's husband. I am also a father, grandfather, and great-grandfather.

Caregiver to my wife is the important and responsible role I carry at this time of my life and over time it has become my occupation. It is somewhat different from the last twenty years of my working life when I was travelling around North America and overseas to Eastern Europe, engaged in public speaking, carrying out the responsibilities of Executive Director for a Christian Mission. Today my occupation is even more important – taking care of Rita's needs. In fact, going further, I would say now, it has become my calling. It certainly has created a real sense of purpose and fulfilment.

I have discovered over the years of caregiving that there has been a certain special bonding which has occurred between us at a much deeper level than would normally occur in a regular day to day marriage relationship. With the daily experience of intimate and personal caring, there has developed a closeness and understanding which would not occur in a non-caring situation. Dependence deepens the love from both sides. I have become Rita's security. Our circumstance has inevitably created an exceptional and close loving relationship.

The relationship between caregiver and the person cared for is unique. It becomes very special over time. I think the closeness which results cannot be experienced in any other way. One lady expressed to me how she saw in her mother a special love and a deeper devotion develop for her dad, as her mother cared for him over many months and years. It probably needs to be experienced to fully appreciate it. I have read many testimonies from people who have struggled with caregiving and found the task very hard but in the end have valued the experience and would do it all over again if necessary.

I believe that what I do for Rita is a reflection of the heart. Actions come from the heart. How we behave, and what we do, originates in the mind which is dictated by how the heart feels. If you love the person you care for, and I mean really love them, then I believe your activity on their behalf will be determined and motivated by that love.

A heart of love will find strength to overcome a myriad of obstacles. It will overlook disappointments. It will overlook faults and imperfections. It will readily forgive mistakes. It will hold you up and keep you going during those bad days, the days you struggle and feel you can no longer go on. Love is stronger than any situation.

In the quiet of the night, I feel so deeply for Rita, understanding the physical predicament she is in and the endlessness of the incapacity. Deep down I have an absolute longing, above all else, to put everything right. But sadly, I cannot bring that about.

Many years ago, 59 to be exact, I made a commitment before a congregation and before God, not only to marry Rita but to care for her regardless of changing circumstances. Regarding the "richer or poorer" clause,

I cannot remember when the "richer" happened, but I can remember the "poorer" period. We worked our way through that time paying one bill while holding on to another, stretching our money as necessary. The "in sickness and in health" clause has affected us both on our journey together, some good healthy times and others not so much. We are now in a permanent "sickness" period within our marriage and a time when our vows have become real in everyday living.

To love and to cherish

It just happens to be this way round; I care for Rita. It could well have been Rita caring for me. However, there was another clause in that commitment which only of late have I come to fully appreciate. It read "to love and to cherish" which is a promise to love, to honour, to hold as valuable and to treasure her. I am sure even when we love, we often overlook the honouring and treasuring. The loving and the cherishing obviously grows in intensity according to the amount of time invested in the relationship, and in caregiving that amount of time is enormous.

In all our marriages as we love and care for our wives, that love gradually deepens over the years. Caregiving takes it to another level. It has only been since the implementation of caregiving that I have come to realize the cherishing aspect of our relationship. To love and to cherish becomes real. I have come to value Rita for who she is and what she means to me. As much as she needs me, I find that I need her. The relationship continues to develop, and the bond deepens. Thus, the caregiving is no longer just duty or even fulfilling a responsibility. It is out of love that I care for Rita as well as fulfilling the commitment and vows made almost six decades ago.

Real love can and does overcome enormous obstacles. It overlooks shortcomings and minimizes other problems. I believe love has bonded us together so that we are stronger as a couple to face life issues as one. Love has helped us to survive through the storms of life. Someone once said, "People die but love never dies!"

Although in one sense my role as caregiver came to me as the natural person to do the job, I discovered that accepting this role and living the part of caregiver out of love, has brought its own incredible rewards. Just having the knowledge that I am helping to relieve the mental turmoil and physical suffering of Rita, cannot be described. To have love and any expression of appreciation returned, is a bonus, and amply provides all the reward one could ever want.

Although Rita has had Parkinson's for over 13 years and she has needed my full-time care for more than half of those years, whatever the future may hold, I will always say it has been a privilege and honour to care for her. Why? Because she is special, she is precious, she is my princess, my Rita.

Part Two

Your Story

My Fellow Caregivers

As you have read through the details of our experience, you might have thought "But you don't know what I have to go through, my situation is far different from yours!" and you are probably right. So many caregivers have differing circumstances, different levels of care required, along with a variety of caring demands. We also deal with people who have vastly different personalities. I empathize with each caregiver for I have become aware of the many difficult challenges each are facing.

When I think about the obstacles and the practical caring implications faced by those tending bedridden people, I feel quite blessed in caring for Rita who, although suffering with a severe incapacity, can still move around with assistance. We also have six friends who are caring for family members who have dementia. They face yet another set of circumstances and experience massive frustration in answering the same question many times a day. Their situations require constant attention because a person suffering with dementia can usually move around freely, often doing things which are unhelpful and sometimes dangerous. My heart goes out to all those whose task is greater than mine, and there are many of you.

Let me say right here that if you are struggling physically and mentally in your caregiving capacity, my word to you is, "Keep going because if I can do it, so can you!" and "You will find it so worthwhile at the end of the day!" Other caregivers have ended their task with "It was hard, but I would not have missed it for anything!"

If you have read everything to this point you have become aware that I do not have all the answers. Even doing the job for years I have not become the expert on caregiving. I have simply shared details of our life and my view of responsibility as caregiver to my wife. Although I might not be the greatest example of caregiving, I have tried to do the best possible job under the circumstances. However, in this section I would like to share with you some of the things I have discovered from practical experience, from reading, and from talking with others. Like me, in this job, you have probably found it true that we never stop learning and are always open to understand how we might do better. So, although what I say may not be very profound, I hope that what you find here will be of help to you in your everyday life of caring.

Help me Understand

This may be obvious, but my first recommendation would be to encourage you to get to know the disease or illness you are dealing with. It will give you a better understanding of what the future will hold. You do not want to be blindsided if things take a turn for the worst. It will help in your mental and physical preparation for what you might have to face in the months, or perhaps years, ahead. Having knowledge and understanding of your situation is invaluable. It gives you the sense of being one step ahead.

I tend to be a person who likes to know as much as I can about any given situation. I find it helps to be informed about the problem or the task I am facing. Parkinson's is a big issue to understand. However, I don't believe you can have too much knowledge of the illness and how it might play out in the future. So, I bought, and read, a 500-page book on Parkinson's. The book is *"The Parkinson's Disease Treatment Book"* which I was told is the Parkinson's Bible. It was written by a world leading Parkinson's specialist, Dr J. Eric Ahlskog, Professor of Neurology at the Mayo Medical School.

You may think buying such a book seems a little over the top. However, it certainly helped me to understand the intricacies of the disease, what to expect, and what to look for. By learning about the illness, I have not been surprised along the way as things have inevitably changed as the illness has progressed. It helps me to accept what I see for what it is and not be surprised by something unexpected. Also having that knowledge has allowed me to be an emotional support to Rita, who could have become disturbed by new symptoms.

The next area of learning was medication. As I have taken care of Rita's medicine from day one, naturally I wanted to know what it was and what it was supposed to be achieving. I also wanted to know how best it should be administered, some with food and some before food. As Rita has medication nine times a day from 7 am to 10.15 pm, I found it essential to ensure that I was giving it correctly.

In talking with other people who are dealing with the same disease, I quickly discovered that you do not compare prescriptions. Every person is different and often treated differently. Because someone else is on a different regimen of medication it does not mean that your doctor has prescribed the wrong dosage or the wrong medication. It is unwise to go down that road. With Parkinson's there is such a range of symptoms that medications and prescriptions differ with each person. I am sure that is the same with other diseases as well.

Right from the beginning I learned as much as I could on the medications and especially how they were to benefit Rita. I found that the more I knew about the

various medications, the more comfortable and knowl-
edgeable I felt when talking with doctors and other
medical personnel. It was even more beneficial when
there was the suggestion of a change. I had sufficient
knowledge to understand why the change and for what
benefit. Just as knowing more about the disability helps
you handle it better, so knowing about the various medi-
cines, gives a sense of confidence in making any adjust-
ments in their administration.

I take the view that the more we know the more effective we will be in our caring. For instance, depression is not
uncommon in Parkinson's patients. Often doctors will
prescribe an anti-depressant along with their Parkinson's
regular medication. With such an insidious disease it is
understandable that for such patients, depression is never
far away. This may be the same with other illnesses.

Those who are being cared for often suffer with constant inner frustration with their situation. A sense of
helplessness and hopelessness can at times pervade their
thinking. It helps to be aware of that. Even without
Parkinson's Rita has always had a disposition which leans
towards anxiousness and because the progression of the
Parkinson's disease could add to any anxiety already
there, it has been wise for me to be cognizant of that. As
Rita's caregiver, to know and understand this, enables me
to purposely give positive input into the situation, thus
helping to avoid anything which might add to the poten-

tiality of depression. This may not apply in your situation. but it is always worthwhile to be sensitive as to how your loved one is feeling towards their incapacity.

I am sure you will excuse me using Parkinson's to illustrate my point but that is what I have dealt with and have come to know, but the principles do apply whatever disease you are dealing with. For instance, I have tried to stay abreast of any new developments in the understanding and treatment of Parkinson's. I have read up on Deep Brain Stimulation and the potential benefits it can bring. This is where electrodes are implanted in the brain for appropriate stimulation. We know of two people who had the operation, both of whom saw an incredible increase in mobility and one particularly in the loss of tremor. The benefits seemed to have lasted about fifteen years. I have also read of other treatments with limited or questionable results.

Whatever you are dealing with, try to learn what is available and what might be coming down the road. I feel it is imperative and responsible to stay informed. In my mind I consider anything that might make my caring better, is essential and necessary for me to check out. I have also discovered that medical professionals seem to appreciate it if you have taken the trouble to keep informed. It also allows you to ask the appropriate and meaningful questions.

I have read several books on caregiving and refer to several websites dedicated to the subject. I would thoroughly recommend it. There is plenty of information available on the internet. It makes sense if you are keen to know how best to do the job. If it makes life easier, then it must be useful and beneficial. I have also tried to learn from others who are doing the same job. There are care-partner meetings online which are places for sharing and learning from others. I take the view that thousands of others have been down the road before me, so I am wide open to hearing how they coped and dealt with various common issues and problems.

The more we understand the less we are surprised. It removes the element of shock. To be prepared for eventualities is a big step forward when dealing with recurrent changes. Stay informed and educate yourself in all aspects. It may seem tedious, but it helps us to understand why we do what we do.

Knowing your loved one

Another big requirement to do our job well is to understand the person we are caring for and by that, I mean to fully appreciate how they think and feel about the situation they find themselves in. They are the ones suffering from the disease and facing the incapacities and limitations day after day. Try to look at life through their eyes. From their disadvantaged viewpoint, things may appear completely different as opposed to your own perspective. They may be mentally frustrated and perhaps overwhelmed. It would be good to know that. It could be something they may not readily share with you without your specifically asking them. It is a case of getting into their mind.

It may take time to discover and understand the emotional suffering they might be experiencing. Listen intently to what they say and how they say it. Respect their thinking. It is they who are living with the disability. Try to learn the specifics of what it is that they struggle with mentally.

I understand that sometimes there is an underlying grieving in their minds, even without their knowledge of it. People with long-term degenerative diseases often have internal regrets. They are grieving for past independence – wishing they had done more, visited more places and achieved more before the onset of their disease. Such thinking can bring about depression as time cannot be regained, nor the opportunities to do the things they had wished. It is so hard for some to recognize and accept that life can never be as it was.

Take note of what bothers them. This may be hard but ask if there is anything you are doing which inadvertently is hurtful or disturbing to them. It may be showing disrespect by talking down to them – something which can so easily be done where communication is difficult. It may be something else quite simple, but your action is being viewed differently from what you intended.

Then there is the pleasant side to this. Investigate what pleases them. What is it that brings pleasure? What do they enjoy? It may be some small aspect which surprises you. There could be something you are overlooking which could brighten their day and bring enjoyment. We must try our utmost to understand what is happening in the mind of our loved one. It will help our level of compassion and sensitivity as we serve and support them.

I have discovered that one of the most pleasurable aspects of the day for Rita is when she is tucked in bed at night, and I am talking or reading to her. I understand this. The struggle of the day is over. Every movement for her is an effort. Every step put forward is so difficult. At that moment she can lay down, relax, and no longer be concerned about the day. There are no more demands upon her. It is her comfort time. It creates a sense of security.

Our Attitude

Respect and dignity are two very important aspects which should be prevalent in our thinking. Both are portrayed by our attitude. Attitude to the job and to the person cared for is critical. We always need to remind ourselves that they are people first and a patient second. We need to always respect them for who they are and for what they have achieved. Everyone has made a difference by being here, both in the family and elsewhere. They have not always been in a wheelchair. At one time they were active and contributed to society around them. We must never treat them as though they have been 'put out to pasture.' They may be dependent on others now but there was a time when that was not the case, and it is important to them that they are treated as a normal regular person and not just as a patient.

Having incapacities does not nullify thinking. Those cared for still have views and opinions. Physical incapacity does not imply a loss of intelligence. They still have feelings and wishes. One area is the area of privacy. Just because they must be dressed or taken to the bathroom, it does not mean that their privacy and dignity is any less important, in fact, it is probably more so. Some are very self-conscious about their "not so young" bodies and care needs to be taken to ensure that is observed.

Usually there is no problem when the spouse is caring for a spouse, but when outside help is used those involved need to be understanding in this area. The person being dressed is entitled to the privacy they desire and as caregiver we are responsible. If you have other people coming in to help with the caring it is necessary to check that they are doing their job in a way which is acceptable to the person cared for. People can do things which are upsetting or embarrassing without even realizing it. For instance, we discovered there are discreet and indiscreet ways to undress someone. We, as caregivers, carry a responsibility to make sure that respect and dignity are not forgotten in the caring process. The comfort of our loved one is always paramount.

If you go out on trips to do shopping or eating out in restaurants, avoid situations which could be embarrassing. A little thoughtfulness goes a long way in ensuring that everything remains within the comfort zone. As caregivers we learn sensitivity from day one and should pick up on anything which is disturbing and deal with it quickly.

Encouragement

There are times when we all need encouragement. So many caregivers work alone, are frustrated, sometimes angry, sad, disappointed, overwhelmed, exhausted and even feel abandoned. You are not abnormal if you are experiencing these emotions or physical feelings. Some feel lonely from being isolated. You may have no family support because there is none to be had. For others you may consider your situation too difficult for friends to step in.

Those who are caring for loved ones with dementia often feel alone, having the added difficulty of not being able to communicate very well with them. Their loved ones are often unable to comprehend what is being said to them and consequently are unable to respond accordingly. Demands on such caregivers are horrendous, continuous, and mentally exhausting. Some also feel extremely sad from seeing their loved one decline and physically overwhelmed by the constant call of the bell or the call of their name.

Encouragement can come from different places. It's so nice to receive an email, phone call or note to remind you that people care for you as the caregiver. Sadly, many people who are not involved in caregiving are unaware of the internal struggle and feelings of loneliness which go with the job, until we share it with them. How often do we put on a brave face and imply that all is well when asked how things are going? Occasionally, it might be wise to be honest and say how you genuinely feel. Let others know just how exhausted you are. If you are experiencing a sense of abandonment perhaps, they should hear that. There are many people who would bring us help and encouragement if they only knew we needed it.

However, a word of warning here. It does depend upon the person to whom you are talking. If you do reveal your honest feelings, remember that you are putting yourself in a vulnerable position, so it would be wise to know well the person with whom you share. Discover their genuineness to help first, and the level of trust. It's important to you.

From day one we have had to recognize that caregiving is a long-haul job, it is a marathon, not a hundred-meter dash or a quick trip around the block. It calls for endless patience, stalwart determination, and perseverance. It is not uncommon for a caregiver to become so overwhelmed as to want to throw in the towel – only to immediately suffer with a sense of guilt for even having such a thought. The physical strain, the emotional turmoil and the constant demands can become seemingly too much to handle. Yet handle it we do. Why? Well, my theory is that we do it because we are motivated by love because love will overcome many obstacles. Love will help you rise from the ashes like the phoenix, many times over.

Enjoy life together

Don't rush through life. By that I mean make the most of the time you have together. It is true that each day has such similarity to the day before and therefore it is easy to get up each morning and think "Same old, same old."We then put ourselves into gear for the day ahead accepting it as being the same as yesterday and the day before. The days may have similar schedules, but we need to treat each day as new and look for that which will cause the day to be different from the day before. It may take some effort and a bit of thinking but attempt to make the day different and look to add variety to the day. This adds interest for you both.

Even if our lives tend to be determined by the demands and needs of each day, we must remain in control by planning and organize the flow of activity if we are to do something different from the day before. I agree with you that this is easier said than done and it is not something I have been good at. This is where jigsaws, cards, Scrabble, or other board games come into play. If you can manage it, a trip out will break up the daily monotony although, as in our case, it might take quite a bit of effort. A little "outside the box" thinking will add some interest and spice to your life.

One of the most essential requirements of our task is to remain flexible. Rarely do things remain the same. By being flexible it enables us to accept changes more readily and easily. There are many things in life which break because they are not flexible, and I guess that goes for people too. Be prepared for any eventuality. Accidents happen without notice. Emergencies can change everything. One minute you can be happy that everything seems to be flowing naturally and normally and the next minute you could be dialing for an ambulance.

Thinking about emergencies it is good to have all necessary paperwork available and handy. List of medications and times they are taken throughout the day. Make a note about allergies. Have a list of the health card number, health insurance details, name, address and telephone number of the private doctor or specialist already involved in the care. If your loved one is taken to hospital suddenly then all this information will be required at a moment's notice.

It is also wise to ensure that all legal papers are up to date. Living with uncertainty of what might be around the corner, it is worth checking that decisions which need to made have been made. We must check things like Power of Attorney or Agreement of Representation just in case others are forced into making decisions for us in the event of our incapacity. It applies to all of us and not just the one being cared for. Make sure wills are up to date and maybe your last wishes, and those of your loved one, have been duly recorded.

The questions need to be asked about choices regarding the last moments of our lives? The question of "Do not resuscitate" needs to be considered or having heroics performed to keep us alive for a few extra hours or maybe days. Some people think that quality of life is more important than quantity. All these aspects need to be discussed. As an aside, I have read that people who choose hospice care for the end of life have a far more peaceable departure than those who are hospitalized and subject to extreme and drastic procedures to keep them alive. All these things call for discussion.

Health matters

Let me throw something in here about health. We have heard it and know the truth of it through and through, that we caregivers should be taking care of our health. One thing I have learned which makes sense, although I have not practiced it much, concerns our breathing. Most of us experience shallow breathing. Any sense of anxiousness will affect our breathing. Constant incorrectly breathing will affect the body. All our major organs need oxygen. I am given to understand that shallow breathing over long periods will deprive vital organs of oxygen and not least the brain, which we all need to operate well in any caregiving situation. It is not an easy thing to remember as we get so tied up in everyday activity but the practice of deep breathing for just ten minutes will do wonders as a coping mechanism in facing overwhelming stress and bothersome issues. Personally, I dislike taking drugs so anything I can do naturally like deep breathing to manage my health I find preferable.

Referring to the aspect of stress, you have probably already found yourself in a state of fatigue or regularly being tired from disturbed nights. The normal stress of

life will always be with us. It is the abnormal and constant stress which we need to avoid. It brings on long-
term health problems. It can creep up on us and show
itself in different ways. It can cause irrational or unwar-
ranted anger or irritability. We can become overly anxious
about the mundane and begin worrying about unrealistic things. We can feel down, sad, or worse, depressed.
We can react unreasonably to minor issues. It can also
accentuate the feeling of being alone, isolated, or overwhelmed. It helps to keep a regular schedule for eating
and sleeping. Try to eat well and sleep well. It may sound
redundant, but it is not if it helps you to cope better.

I read that it is not uncommon for many caregivers without any religious connection, to seek comfort
in prayer or spiritual counsel. That makes sense because
talking over the situation with an objective party can do
wonders for the mind. To get an outside perspective on
your situation often brings a dimension not seen before
and sometimes provides answers which have been over-
looked. To have a trusted friend with whom you can share
your concerns, is invaluable. Such support is immeasur-
able.

In thinking about support don't forget the groups
that have been set up in your community to provide help.
It is surprising but, in these groups, you discover others
who are dealing with the same issues and facing the
same problems you are. You quickly understand that you

are not the only one struggling with various obstacles. Support groups are good for the caregiver and the person cared for. There are places also which offer day care for the incapacitated, thus offering a few hours of respite for the caregiver. They provide the mental and emotional support needed. We all benefit from the confidence and assurance that we are not in this alone. I once read that we fail to seek help to our own detriment – a lesson I am still learning.

One of the most important aspects of preparation is for the caregiver to create an outside interest. Why? Because once separation happens – and it inevitably will – there will be a huge void to fill. If you are in a 24/7 care situation then there is a busyness which suddenly is not there. I have thought much about this for myself wondering how I would occupy that time. Fortunately, I have real interests in reading, writing, and collecting obsolete British and Canadian banknotes. I also taught myself to play the organ which I enjoy.

It is critical to think about this so that your mind can easily adjust to something in which you have a real interest. Some people have taken to art, learning how to draw or paint. Some have taken up learning how to play a musical instrument. Others have turned their attention to more practical hands-on hobbies such as quilting or crocheting. Another area of very high interest today is memoir writing, either personal and biographical or family memoirs. Endless hours can be spent in research in any one of these areas. If you have an interest in collecting, then there are coins, stamps, obsolete comics, and antiques. Any one of these things will bring a sense of purpose and add interest to your day.

One of the greatest rewards we get from doing this job is simply to know how much we are helping our loved one. It is always an expression of love. Don't even wonder as to whether it is being appreciated or not. We are doing the job not for what we get out of it but to serve and be a blessing and a life support for those for whom we care. So be encouraged. It's alright for you to think that you are the best qualified person to do the job because you probably are. To know what you are doing and achieving for your loved one is more than adequate reward. Let me again quote other caregivers who finish the journey by saying "It was hard work, but I am glad I did it. It was so worthwhile."

It is common knowledge that caregivers become overwhelmed with the task and if you are one of them, let me encourage you. Try to rise above it and think of the humorous quotation, from Mark Twain, "I have been through some terrible things in my life, some of which actually happened."

I am sure you agree with me that none of us is perfect and never will be, but we do what we can with the ability we have, regardless of the sometimes-untenable circum-stances we find ourselves in.

So, my fellow Caregivers. Keep working, keep helping, keep loving and be encouraged. Even if it is not always expressed, your efforts are deeply appreciated. You are important because you play an important role. At this moment you are indispensable. You are the pillar which provides critical support. One day you will have a sense of comfort and satisfaction in the knowledge that you did what you could, you did your best. That is all that can be expected of you.

Books Referenced:

Chapter 6.
Finding grace in the face of Dementia by Dr. John Dunlop.
Published by Crossway, 2017.

Chapter 7.
The Year of Magical Thinking by Joan Didion.
Published by Harper Collins, 2012.

Books you may find helpful:

Passages in Caregiving by Gail Sheehy.
Published by HarperCollins Publishers, 2010

Caregiving for Parkinson's Disease by Lianna Marie.
Published by Lianna Marie, 2016

A Promised Kept by Robertson McQuilkin.
Published by Tyndale Press, 1998

Caregiving: A privilege, not a prison by June Hunt.
Published by Aspire Press, 2017

A word from the author...

If you have enjoyed reading this book and have found it meaningful, would you encourage others to read it also. You can do this by kindly going to Amazon.com, find the book and leave a sentence or two as a review? That would be very helpful, and I would appreciate it immensely. Let me thank you in advance for doing that.

John Murray.

To connect with the author:
email: murray150@fastmail.fm
twitter: @AuthorJMurray
facebook.com/AuthorJohnMurray
website: http://www.jmurray.ca

To order more copies of this book, find books by other Canadian authors, or make inquiries about publishing your own book, contact PageMaster at:

PageMaster Publication Services Inc.
11340-120 Street, Edmonton, ABT5G 0W5
books@pagemaster.ca
780-425-9303

catalogue and e-commerce store
PageMasterPublishing.ca/Shop

About the Author

John has been married to his wife Rita for almost 60 years. They have two children, five grandchildren and two great-grandchildren. Originally from the U.K. they now reside in White Rock, British Columbia, on the west coast of Canada.

Educated in England, John went on to study theology in Birmingham, U.K. and in Toronto, Canada. His life experience has been in business, in journalism, in pastoral ministry and overseas missions.

For the last twenty years before retiring he served as the Executive Director for Eurovangelism Canada, a mission working in Eastern Europe. He travelled extensively from Russia in the north to Albania in the south. Some of the stories in the book *Miracles: Coincidence or Divine Intervention* are from his days travelling in Eastern Europe.

His many years of speaking engagements took him to ten countries which included Canada, the United States, the United Kingdom, Europe and the Caribbean.

Since retiring in 2006 John has concentrated on his writing. *It's All About Love* is his fifth book.